Should Medial Care
Be Rationed by Age?

Should Medical Care Be Rationed by Age?

Edited by
Timothy M. Smeeding
with
Margaret P. Battin
Leslie P. Francis
Bruce M. Landesman

ROWMAN & LITTLEFIELD
PUBLISHERS

362.19897
S559

ROWMAN & LITTLEFIELD

Published in the United States of America in 1987
by Rowman & Littlefield, Publishers
(a division of Littlefield, Adams & Company)
81 Adams Drive, Totowa, New Jersey 07512

The articles herein were originally presented at the conference
"Health Care Rationing Among the Elderly: Aging, Ethics,
Politics, and Economics," at the University of Utah, September 13
and 14, 1985.

Library of Congress Cataloging-in-Publication Data

Should medical care be rationed by age?

Based on a conference held at the University of Utah, Sept.
13–14, 1985, sponsored by the University of Utah Health
Technology and Environment Research Group.

Includes bibliographies and index.

1. Aged—Medical care—United States—Cost effectiveness—
Congresses. 2. Aged—Medical care—United States—Moral and
ethical aspects—congresses. 3. Aged—Medical care—Cost
effectiveness—congresses. 4. Aged—Medical care—Moral and
ethical aspects—congresses. I. Smeeding, Timothy M.
II. University of Utah. Health Technology and Environment Research
Group. [DNLM: 1. Delivery of Health Care—economics—
congresses. 2. Ethics, Medical—congresses. 3. Health
Resources—supply and distribution—congresses.
4. Health Services for the Aged—supply and distribution—
congresses. 5. Policy Making—congresses.
WT 30 S559 1985]
RA564.8.S53   1987   362.1'9897'00973   86-15440
ISBN 0-8476-7521-1

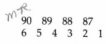

90   89   88   87
6   5   4   3   2   1

Printed in the United States of America

Contents

Tables and Figures

Acknowledgments

THE ARTICLES in this volume were originally presented at the September 1985 Conference, "Health Care Rationing Among the Elderly: Aging, Ethics, Politics and Economics," sponsored by the University of Utah Health Technology and Environment Research Group under the general coordination of Timothy M. Smeeding, Director of the University's Division of Social Science Research in the Center for Public Affairs and Administration.

A number of people at the University of Utah deserve special thanks for helping make the conference a success: in particular, Howard Ball, Dean of the College of Social and Behavioral Science, the prime financial sponsor; Ted Wilson, Director of the Hinckley Institute of Politics; Cecil M. Samuelson, Dean of the College of Medicine; Margaret Dimond, Director of the University of Utah Gerontology Program; and an anonymous donor who proffered financial assistance. Rosalie Webb, Jolaine Randall, and Jeanne Ward handled the conference arrangements. Nancy Robinson and her staff at the Rustler Lodge, Alta, Utah, provided wonderful food, lodging, and weather.

We are grateful to Don E. Detmer, Vice President for Health at the University of Utah; Richard D. Lamm, Governor of Colorado; and David N. Sundwall, staff physician to the U.S. Senate Committee on Labor and Human Resources, who addressed the conference; to the contributors for their prompt revisions; and to other conference participants for their helpful comments and suggestions, many of which are reflected in the revised papers and in the summary and assessment chapter.

The views expressed in the book are solely those of the authors and commentators, and should not be construed as representing the official policies of the University of Utah, or those of the institutions with which individual authors or commentators are affiliated.

T.M.S., M.P.B., L.P.F., and B.R.L.

Conference Participants

Howard Ball, University of Utah

Margaret P. Battin, University of Utah

Gary Bryner, Brigham Young University

John Bunker, M.D., Stanford Medical Center

Thomas H. Caine, M.D., University of Utah

John Collette, University of Utah

Suzanne Dandoy, M.D., Utah State Health Department

Don E. Detmer, M.D., University of Utah

Margaret Dimond, University of Utah

Jan Eldred, Henry J. Kaiser Family Foundation

Steve Eraker, M.D., Veterans Administration Medical Center

John Francis, University of Utah

Leslie Francis, University of Utah

Gary Gillund, University of Utah

Gerald Goodenough, M.D., University of Utah

David Green, M.D., University of Utah

F. Ted Hebert, University of Utah

John Horn, University of Denver

Charles Hughes, University of Utah

Dennis Jahnigen, M.D., Veterans Administration Medical Center, Denver

Mary Ann Johnson, University of Utah

Richard D. Lamm, Governor, State of Colorado

Bruce Landesman, University of Utah

Stephen Long, Congressional Budget Office

Robert N. Mayer, University of Utah

James Nickell, University of Colorado

S. Jay Olshansky, Argonne National Laboratory

Stephen Reynolds, University of Utah

Susan Sample, University of Utah

Cecil Samuelson, M.D., University of Utah

John Short, Independent Consultant in Health Care

Peter Singer, Utah Health Cost Management Foundation

Timothy M. Smeeding, University of Utah

David Sundwall, M.D., U.S. Senate Committee on Labor and Human Resources

Keith Tolman, M.D., University of Utah

Robert Utzinger, American Association of Retired Persons

Daniel Wikler, University of Wisconsin

Ted Wilson, University of Utah

Peter Windt, University of Utah

Foreword

Ethical Health Care
for the Elderly: Are We
Cheating Our Children?

Richard D. Lamm

It is difficult to judge whether and in what form ideas generated by students and scholars are translated into action by public policy-makers. Having served in the academic community, I know that this is cause for frustration. There is an old Greek proverb, "To know all to ask is to know half." The tough questions about health care for the elderly will not go away. By asking them, we perform a function that is invaluable. Sometimes it is difficult to see how these ideas take shape in the minds of the voters, but they do.

Ethical care for the elderly raises broad questions. Public policy thinkers and practitioners must look at the issue of health care for the elderly in relation to other social institutions, and in relation to other needy populations. This issue cannot be understood and dealt with responsibly if we examine it in isolation.

I am haunted by the fear that we are being unethical toward our children. I think that $200 billion deficits are profoundly unethical. One dollar borrowed today, at 10 percent interest, paid off over the next 30 years, eventually costs $17.00 to pay back. This year's deficit alone, paid back over the next 30 years, becomes a $3 trillion obligation on our children. Our children, in my opinion, are the gypped generation. At some point they are going to come to us and say, "What have you done to us? You're not paying your own way. You're not making the hard decisions. You are passing them on to us." That we are passing these decisions on is wrong. I believe very strongly that the questions about *any* public dollar—whether it is spent for the elderly or for children—must be examined in a broad context.

If we look at the hard choices within the context of a congressional budget, for example, we are guided by yesterday's ethic of an expanding economic pie. But the financial reality that we must come to grips with is that the economic pie is static. These two ideas have not yet converged, but inevitably they must. We are going to have to make hard choices. To me, the only honest political platform is, "I'm going to raise your taxes; I'm going to cut your benefits; and I'm going to reform your systems." This is what a $200 billion deficit means.

In considering the way we care for our elderly, I start out not with health care but with pension systems. In the total context of caring for the elderly, we have systems that are not well focused. We cannot allow government employees, e.g., to retire in their thirties, with indexed pensions, with health benefits extending into the indefinite future, and have a sane budget. In the military retirement system, the average enlisted man retires at 39, and the average officer retires at 43. Twenty-six percent of the people that retire on military pensions retire while they are still in their thirties. If a veteran took a bullet in Normandy, I think we ought to pay whatever it costs to make him well or to keep him comfortable to the end of his life. If he fell off a bar stool in Hoboken, our obligations to him are different.

Federal Civil Service pensions are similarly lavish. Four out of five people who receive federal Civil Service pensions also receive some other pension at the same time. Seventy percent of them collect Social Security. One out of four is allowed to retire on disability. We must focus the systems that we have in these areas and examine how they are affected by our burgeoning health care costs.

Ultimately, we will have to scrutinize the Social Security system. The Social Security system is the most successful antipoverty program in our history. It is a terrific program, but it is also an intergenerational tax. We must reexamine it if our goal is ethical care for both our elderly and our children. When 25 percent of the people who receive Social Security have other retirement income of over $50,000 a year, we have an ethical obligation to ask, "Does it make any sense to tax the working poor to send money to retired persons with an already more-than-adequate income?" What I refer to is Lamm's "insult everybody a little bit" plan. But we must ask these questions.

The demographic future of America is going to force us to examine these issues. Linus in Peanuts says, "There's no issue too big you can't run away from it." Our forefathers were able to make more generous decisions when America had a trade surplus, and when we didn't have the federal deficits we have now.

Our fathers receive fourteen times what they paid in on their Social

Security. Our children, says the Congressional Budget Office, will be lucky if they get back 73 percent of what they pay into the Social Security system. The broad, inclusive context within which responsible decisions can be made mandates a series of Hobson's choices. We can wish that they would go away, that we lived in a world that did not have deficits, and that America was economically supreme; but that is not the reality that we face. On the contrary, we face an America that is falling increasingly behind in the economic race. Wherever we look, our systems are out of control.

Health care relates to these other systems. The one inescapable lesson for one who balances a budget is that health care today is interfering with other social obligations. Governor Kean of New Jersey, in a phrase that I wish I had coined, calls health care the "Pac Man of his budget." It indiscriminately eats up all his flexibility. Consequently, laudable projects are shelved. Since 1950, health care has been rising at 10.6 percent per year. No set of expenditures can rise faster than the GNP forever.

Our societal values, then, include more than just good health care for the elderly. How do we retool America? How do we reform our educational system? The relationship of health care costs to other programs is fascinating. In 1950, government spending for health care was 45 percent of what we spent on education. In 1984, it was equal to all the money spent by the federal government on education. Our whole fiscal system is tilting toward health care. This trend cannot continue if we want our children to have jobs.

Even within the artificially circumscribed context of the health care system, we are not allocating our resources wisely. In the spring of 1985, I spent a week in England looking at the English health care system. We spend $1500 per capita on health care, the English spend $400 per capita, Singapore spends $200 per capita, and the mortality and morbidity rates of all of these countries are the same.

While mortality and morbidity alone are not adequate yardsticks by which to measure a good health care system, nonetheless, there seems to be an intriguing inverse correlation between the number of physicians in a society and the society's overall level of health. West Germany has the most doctors per capita, and they are the unhealthiest. Japan has the smallest number of doctors per capita, and they are the healthiest. The biggest strides in health care history have resulted from doctors or hospitals—refrigeration, vaccination, and sanitation. Public health professionals are the unheralded heroes. Yet, it is estimated that the United States has spent more money on health care in the last six months of peoples' lives than the gross national product of Bangladesh. It is clear to me that we are misallocating much of our health resources.

Part of the problem is our attitude towards technology. We seem to think rather simplistically that more is better. Victor Fuchs says, "The desire of the engineer to build the best bridge, or the physician to practice in the best equipped hospital is understandable." However, to the extent that the monotechnic person fails to recognize the claims of competing priorities, his advice is likely to be a poor guide to social policy.

Another part of the problem is our attitude towards death. Ivan Illich says, "The medicalization of our society has brought the epoch of natural death to an end." Western man has lost the right to preside at his act of dying. Health or the autonomous power to cope has been expropriated down to the very last breath. Death and dying are the last taboo. This is certainly true with politicians, I can guarantee.

We neither can nor should want to defeat death. Death is part of life. The tragedy of life is not death; it is dying unfulfilled, not having loved, without accomplishments. This is a very sensitive subject, as I have found out; but it is a subject that must be discussed.

Quite simply, we may not now be making ethical decisions in the treatment of the elderly and the terminally ill. Decision-makers do not look at what is really good for the patient, but what will stand up to a lawsuit. The law hangs over us like a sword of Damocles. The conflict, in fact, often lies between the best treatment you can give to the elderly and what you actually can do technologically. Actions, like the recent indictment in California of two physicians who discontinued a life support system with the wife's consent, sent shock waves throughout the medical world. Such events make it more difficult for us to make ethical decisions for the terminally ill. The result is decisions that favor more technology and the protection of the doctor from the law, not the benefit of the patient. The doctor is concerned with the possibility of a malpractice suit, bad publicity, or a stain on his or her career for failing to order technological intervention at the last stages of a patient's illness. For the patient, this is not treatment; it is torture.

Certainly we should spend more money and expend more effort to enhance everyone's chance of attaining a normal life span. We should also strive to increase everyone's chance for a normal quality of life. There are profound differences between—on the one hand, a hip operation, a cornea transplant, or other procedures that add much to the quality of life of a senior, and on the other, efforts to keep alive a stroke victim who is comatose and on a life support system, or the victim of dementia in its final stages.

One doctor, in the *New England Journal of Medicine* wrote, "My personal experience in the practice of neurology over the past twenty years is [that] there's a widespread refusal to acknowledge suffering and degradation experienced by helpless people permanently maintained on life support systems. The American health care system breeds a mentality of turning away from this consideration, perhaps because it does not acknowledge the reality that there is a time to die."

Karl Barth said, "Life is no second God, therefore the respect due to it cannot rival the reverence owed to God."

Two doctors recently stated in the *New England Journal of Medicine*, "The emphasis on mortality statistics as a measure of medical care has tended to obscure the fact that most of the time and effort of practicing physicians is devoted to improving the life of the patient— adding life to our years, not meaningless years to our lives. The real enemies are disease, discomfort, disability, fear, and anxiety—not death."

I very much believe in these statements.

A society that borrows from its grandchildren, fails to retool its economic system, neglects its educational system, and pours our limited resources into extending a few days of life at great suffering to the patient, is a profoundly unethical society. When we start using machines that do not cure or heal, that do not prolong life, but merely extend dying, then we are trying in vain to stop the irreversible. We have abdicated our role as ethical human beings. We are making sacrifices to that secular god "technology" that are profoundly wrong. Our priorities are misplaced. If we do not succeed in reorienting them, we will indeed cheat our children and generations to come.

Should Medial Care
Be Rationed by Age?

1

Introduction

Leslie P. Francis
Timothy M. Smeeding

WE ARE AN AGING SOCIETY. According to the United States Bureau of the Census, in 1960, just before the introduction of Medicare, 9.2 percent of the population were over age 65 and .5 percent fell into the group we now call the "old-old," the cohort aged 85 and above.[1] By 1980, the percentage of the elderly in the population, like the percentage of gross national product devoted to health care, had topped 10 percent; 11.3 percent were over 65 and 1 percent were over 85. The census bureau projects that by the year 2000, 13 percent of the population will be over 65, and 1.8 percent will be over 85. The 85 and over group is the fastest growing age group in the United States today and will continue to be so at least until the year 2000. By the year 2050, 21.8 percent will be over 65 and 5.2 percent over 85.

These demographic shifts in the American population are a combined result of increases in life expectancy and decreases in the birth rate. Thus, they represent both an increase in actual numbers in the older age cohorts and a declining increase in numbers in the lower cohorts. These demographic changes can be expected to have major economic, social, and political effects, especially in the eight states in which over half the elderly live: California, New York, Florida, Pennsylvania, Texas, Illinois, Ohio, and Michigan. The very elderly, for example, are more likely to be female, to live alone, to rely on social security or assets rather than on earned income, and to spend a higher percentage of their incomes on necessities. In general, the elderly are being encouraged to retire at earlier ages, and once retired, tend not to engage in economically productive or voluntary work.[2] They are less likely to move (except to the sun belt); to live in large, single-family dwellings; or to purchase consumer goods.[3] For our purposes, perhaps most importantly of all, they are less likely to be healthy and more likely to need medical care or home health services, especially as the newly retired elderly in their 60s become the "old-old" in their 80s.

The medical care needed by the elderly, moreover, is likely to be different from the medical care needed at younger ages. The elderly are more likely to suffer from chronic or disabling conditions than their younger counterparts. More than four-fifths of those over age 65 suffer from at least one chronic condition including arthritis, hypertension or heart disease, hearing or vision impairment, orthopedic conditions such as osteoporosis, or sinusitis. Estimates are that in 1985 some 5.2 million of those aged 65 and above required some assistance or special aid to maintain independence because of a chronic condition, and these numbers are expected to double within the next 40 years. Mental health needs of the elderly are more likely to include cognitive impairment, such as Alzheimer's disease, and are especially likely to result in nursing home care. In 1985, approximately 5 percent of the elderly were in nursing homes on any given day, although these figures rise to nearly 20 percent for the oldest old, those over age 85.

In addition to chronic care, the elderly are more likely to need acute care than the young. The elderly are hospitalized about twice as often, stay longer despite the shorter stay incentives introduced by the prospective payment system for Medicare patients, and are more likely to be readmitted within a year.[4] They also visit physicians and take prescription medications more frequently than the young. These figures rise sharply as well within the population over age 65.

These changes in health care utilization by the elderly point to increased health care costs in the future. Over one-third of the nation's expenditures on health care now benefit the elderly. Per capita spending on health care for the elderly has been growing at a rate of nearly 13 percent per annum over the last 15 years. About half of these expenditures are paid by Medicare. Moreover, almost one-third of all Medicare expenditures are concentrated on care of the dying in the final year of life.[5]

Thus, it is clear that we as a society will increasingly face the effects of future demographic change, particularly in health care utilization. Far less clear, however, is what these effects will be; what choices we will have available to us; and how we, as a society, will go about making these choices. The papers in this volume, initially presented at a conference at the University of Utah in September 1985, and revised for this volume, address some aspect of more precise questions. Will the graying of the population be accompanied by increased morbidity or changing notions of the quality of life? How, if at all, should health care for the elderly be publicly financed? Should we encourage the view that there is a time to die, as much as we now attempt to prolong life to the utmost? And how should a democratic society go about making decisions on these complex issues?

Foreword

We begin with a challenge from Governor Lamm. What would we sacrifice if we gave a blank check for health care to the elderly? What are we sacrificing if we continue with current cost cutting efforts, but do not look more deeply at transfer payments up the age scale? The Governor contends that, if we must rely on large deficits to finance health care, retirement benefits, or pensions, we are cheating the next generation. He suggests some solutions: higher taxes, a hard look at pensions that appear to be mere windfalls, and acceptance of the inevitability of the dying process. Even these measures, however, may leave us with hard intergenerational choices depending on the eventual needs of our elderly citizens.

Mortality and Morbidity

The first two chapters deal with important issues about the potential health needs of an aging population. In "The Fourth Stage of the Epidemiologic Transition: Declining Mortality in Advanced Ages," S. Jay Olshansky and A. Brian Ault argue that the significant gains in life expectancy now being made are the result of increased longevity among older age cohorts, indeed, in each of the age cohorts over 65. This increase among older cohorts stands in sharp contrast to earlier gains, which were achieved mostly by declines in death rates from infectious and parasitic disease earlier in the life cycle. It is accompanied by marked changes in the causes of death, so that at present, three-fourths of all deaths at advanced ages occur as a result of degenerative diseases. Moreover, increases in life span among the elderly are accomplished by a postponement of the ages at which degenerative diseases tend to kill, not by further changes in the causes of death. A failure to understand this epidemiological process, Olshansky suggests, may have led demographers to underestimate projections of the numbers of the elderly in the population of the next century.

Olshansky also hypothesizes that these shifts will have important implications for the health care system, depending on their effects on morbidity among the elderly. The most likely possibility is that morbidity and mortality will shift to later ages, but even so, there will be an absolute increase in morbidity as greater numbers survive to older ages. In commenting on Olshansky's paper, Dr. Suzanne Dandoy suggests that much of the gain in longevity among the elderly may have resulted from increased access to health care through Medicare. If so, efforts to ration health care among the elderly may retard the longevity gains Olshansky predicts. Moreover, if rationing is concentrated on diagnostic or preventive services, the result may be increasing morbidity among the elderly as well.

One especially important factor in assessing the health needs of the elderly is cognitive status. In "Memory Processes in the Aged," Gary Gillund tackles the crucial question of cognitive functioning, whether memory steadily declines with advancing age. He argues that it does not. Memory is a complex of processes that entails encoding information within a knowledge structure, storing, and retrieving it. According to Gillund, age alone does not appear to cause knowledge structure to become less functional, although the content of the structures may change with the result that instruments designed for younger age cohorts are not as accurate in measuring performance by the elderly. While information processing does appear to decline with age, this decline may be offset by functional knowledge structures. Gillund notes that individualized differences are greater among the elderly than among younger cohorts, and may be expected to increase with the longevity projections made by Olshansky. The health status of the older old is particularly likely to influence individual variation in memory function because of the effects on memory of chronic conditions such as hypertension, although some of the variation may be reduced by improved medical care. Alzheimer's disease may be cause for deep concern. As deaths are postponed to later ages, rates of Alzheimer's or other dementias may increase sharply, bringing with them sharp declines in cognitive functioning among the elderly who contract them.

If memory and other cognitive processes exhibit significant changes among the elderly, their capacities for ethical and political citizenship may also change radically. John Horn draws out some of the implications of Gillund's findings on this topic. For example, our beliefs—largely unexamined—about the declining capacities of the elderly underlie mandatory retirement policies. Horn argues that both Gillund's data and his own show that there is good scientific reason to question hasty generalizations about cognitive decline in the elderly. If contribution to the general social good is fundamental to the allocation of social resources, the cognitive status of the elderly is not, by itself, sufficient to support age rationing of jobs, health care, or other social goods. The elderly have acquiesced to practices, such as mandatory retirement, that consign them to the status of expendable luxuries. Horn concludes with a potential mandate to action: that if the elderly rest on their capacities, they do not deserve the resource transfers they currently receive. Horn's position suggests another answer to Governor Lamm's challenge—contributions by the elderly themselves as a way to offset the costs of their care. It also, ironically, suggests a vicious cycle in the rationing foreseen by Dr. Dandoy: that failure by the elderly to use their capacities may undermine their claims on the very social resources, such as health care, that help to keep these capacities going.

A Time to Die

Horn's ethical claim that the distribution of social resources should be based on contribution to the social good, however, is disputed by many moral philosophers. In "Age-Rationing and the Just Distribution of Health Care: Is There a Time to Die?," Margaret Battin explores a different approach to the just distribution of health care, using John Rawls's and Norman Daniels's model for the choice of principles of distributive justice and distributive institutions. In brief, the model asks what principles we would adopt were we rational but ignorant of the likely consequences of the policies for our own lives. Rationing health care is just with this approach, if it would be chosen by individuals who cannot predict their own eventual health needs. Daniels has argued that age rationing of health care may indeed be the result of such rational but impartial choice, because it represents the decision to shift health resources to efforts to ensure a normal life span rather than delayed mortality for the few. Thus, age rationing is best regarded as a reallocation of resources within the life cycle, rather than a redistribution from the old to the young.

The thrust of Battin's paper is to question the rationality of this reallocation within the life cycle. Like Dandoy, Battin points out that the effect of rationing health care among the elderly may be increased periods of morbidity; a decision not to treat a particular condition will not magically wave the patient out of existence. Rational choosers contemplating rationing policy must be aware of the degradation it may cause as well as the costs it may save. If so, Battin argues, they may find rationing alone worse than other alternatives. One such alternative, of particular interest to Battin, is combining rationing with support for decisions by the elderly to terminate treatment and to end their lives voluntarily at the point of pronounced and irreversible increases in morbidity. To be sure, talk of encouraging even voluntary euthanasia among the elderly is shocking, as reactions to Governor Lamm's suggestion that there is "a time to die" attest. But Battin's point is that it is crueler still to ration health care in a manner that consigns the elderly to a tortuous morbidity. Our preferred choices in answering Governor Lamm's challenge, therefore, may be either to fund health care more fully among the elderly, or to couple rationing with institutions that bring mortality and morbidity together voluntarily.

In his comments on Battin's essay, Daniel Wikler congratulates Battin on her courage to pose trenchant and unsettling arguments that cannot be ignored, but then argues that her conclusions do not follow from her premises. He first accepts Battin's contractarian approach, but then argues that it does not imply that justice requires us to encourage voluntary euthanasia at the time of approaching terminal illness. Suicide at the onset of terminal illness should not be seen as a duty, according to Wikler, because it may be neither prudent nor recommended. If the elderly decline to make use of health care resources that are offered them, as in Governor Lamm's notion of a time to die, then so be it. However, Wikler's just society cannot deny these resources to the old and sick if they want and need them. In the end, Wikler argues, the problem of age rationing is a political, not a philosophical problem, and therefore deserves a political answer.

Quality of Life

Before turning to politics, John Collette and Peter T. Windt in "Medical Decision-Making, Dying, and Quality of Life," turn their attention to the issue of dying and the elderly, this time asking the elderly (including spouses), and their children and physicians, under what conditions they would want to forego life-extending measures and, instead, die. They address the question of how participants in medical decisions about elderly patients view the importance of quality of life in making life-extending decisions. The authors make it clear that they are not concerned with actual ex post facto quality of life, but rather with the role played by the decision-maker's perception of what quality will be. Collette and Windt obtained survey information on five conditions that seriously affect quality of life: bed confinement, respirator dependency, incontinence, entering a skilled nursing facility, and constant pain.

The findings indicate that the first two conditions were perceived as least acceptable by all three groups, but that elderly persons hypothetically facing such conditions themselves were somewhat less accepting than were spouses or children (middle-aged persons), and especially less accepting than physicians. Based on these analyses, Collette and Windt argue that nonpatients will often perceive the degree of threat to life quality differently from patients, and therefore, the medical decisions made on a patient's behalf might not always conform to the patient's wishes. In particular, their results suggest that individuals are more likely to impose conditions on others which they might not be willing to accept themselves, and that it is more likely that an unacceptable life will be prolonged than an acceptable life terminated.

While these observations do not answer the normative question of what role one's own perception of quality of life should play in medical decision-making, they do suggest that if such perceptions should play an important role, the medical decision-making process may be seriously flawed. Others may choose to expend medical resources to prolong a life for someone whose own decision might have been different. Collette and Windt end with several additional research questions that need to be answered to understand the dynamics of medical decision-making more fully.

Dr. Dennis Jahnigen, a physician and chief of a geriatric medical center, responds thoughtfully to these arguments. Jahnigen readily admits and even cites studies that show that there is considerable concern and difference of opinion among physicians concerning preservation of life in cases in which it does not seem to be consistent with the patient's values, preferences, or choices. However, Jahnigen raises important questions and caveats about the techniques that Collette and Windt use to address their questions. In particular, he is uncomfortable with asking hypothetical questions of elderly persons in good health when the answers to these questions might be quite different should the elderly individual come face to face with an imminent situation that will reduce life quality. Lack of prior experience with any of these conditions is another problem that might lead to decisions based on misinformation. For instance, Jahnigen asks how many of the respondents realize that one-third or more of all nursing home residents regain their health sufficiently to return to their homes, when the common public perception is that no one comes back alive after entering such a facility? Jahnigen makes the salient point that physicians are most likely to have had prior experience with each of these conditions, and are, therefore, more likely to assess them realistically. Certainly Jahnigen, Collette, and Windt agree that future work is needed to compare the degree to which actual decisions conform to hypothetical decisions, and that future physicians need to undergo an educational process that will better prepare them to make such decisions on an individualized patient basis. Jahnigen ends his comment by outlining one such process.

British Injustice?
John G. and Leslie P. Francis, in "Rationing of Health Care in Britain: An Ethical Critique of Public Policy-making," treat Wikler's observa-

tion that health care rationing among the elderly is a political decision by exploring age rationing under the British National Health Science (NHS). The recent well-known book by Henry Aaron and William B. Schwartz[6] suggests that the British experience may prove prescient for health policy in the United States. Francis and Francis, however, challenge this observation and argue that the type of rationing that currently takes place in the British NHS is neither just nor ethical.

They begin by pointing out, as does Smeeding in the following chapter, that political (and individual) rationing of health care takes place all the time. However, political rationing is just only if, in fact: 1. it is made with the participation of those whose interests are at stake; 2. it is made with explicit awareness that rationing was at issue; and 3. alternatives are available should those whose interests are at stake disagree with the social consensus. They go on to argue that none of these conditions are present when NHS nephrologists choose, for instance, not to undertake kidney dialysis for older patients. Ironically, they argue, the NHS was established to equalize access to health care, not to permit a bureaucracy with autonomous physicians to decide who gets what, without public discourse.

Perhaps more interesting, argue the Francises, are the emerging data that indicate that health care rationing in Britain has, in fact, been largely based on age criteria. When faced with a less than fully funded NHS, the controlling physicians chose to ration care largely by age, without public debate. The Francises close their paper with the comment that when there are hard choices to be made, it matters how they are made and how those choices are communicated to the public.

In his Comments, James W. Nickel argues that rationing, if used in the Aaron and Schwartz sense of less than one could conceivably need, is a misnomer. He prefers to treat medical care like any other important but expensive good: one cannot expect to have a political right to as much as one could conceivably need. Nickel believes that political decisions about how much service to provide are needed, but it should not be assumed that all possible services will be provided to each and every citizen.

Nickel agrees with the Francises that public policy must attend to both procedural and substantive aspects of service level reductions, but then questions how to implement such choices politically, and at what level of delivery the hard choices should be made. Where the Francises criticize the policy of allowing local and regional physicians the flexibility of making these choices given a budget from the central government, Nickel argues that such a decentralized system is preferable when medical needs vary across regions.

Coverage and Payment

In the final chapter, "Artificial Organs, Transplants and Long-Term Care for the Elderly: What's Covered? Who Pays?," Timothy M. Smeeding, an economist, suggests that rationing of health care be seen as the process of setting equitable limits on health care availability. He argues that rationing of health care for the elderly involves answering two questions: 1. *What* services should be entitled, i.e., publicly financed?, and 2. *Who* should pay for this health care in general and for entitlements in particular? Two examples of costly health care procedures, entitlement to "spare parts" (artificial and human organ transplants) and to long-term care, are used to illustrate these principles.

Smeeding argues that while certain types of organ transplants and artificial organ implants are proving cost effective, others, particularly those that primarily extend life like the artificial heart, are still a long way from being cost effective. The elderly is one of the least likely groups to receive such treatments should rationing of health care resources become a reality, argues Smeeding, since the cost of treating them is greater, and improvement in quality and quantity of life is less than for other age groups. Smeeding also evaluates long-term care subsidies beyond current Medicaid and Medicare payment practices from a health care rationing point of view. He argues that responsibilities concerning who is covered for what procedures, and who pays, need to be carefully articulated before policy changes are enacted.

A case is made for excluding cost-ineffective treatments that are primarily life extending from Medicare coverage on two grounds: 1. the elderly should bear more financial responsibility for such treatments because society at large benefits less from extending their lives; and 2. the elderly bear more financial responsibility because, by and large, today's elderly can afford to do so. Several mechanisms for self-finance of such treatments by the elderly are suggested by Smeeding in closing.

Epilogue

The final task of summarizing the papers falls to John Bunker and Bruce Landesman. They identify seven major themes or issues:

1. An increasing need for health care among the elderly;
2. How far can we go towards meeting that need if waste is eliminated?

3. The effectiveness of new health care institutions in meeting those needs;
4. The impact of such institutions on the physician-patient relationship and the quality of care;
5. The possibility of age discrimination;
6. The role of the public in health-care decision-making;
7. The moral implications of letting people die.

Bunker and Landesman conclude that the major question of this volume remains unsettled; can we ration health care by age—if we must—sensibly, morally, and justly?

Notes

1. Unless otherwise identified, data in this discussion are drawn from the U.S. Senate Special Committee on Aging. Aging America: Trends and Projections, 1985–86 edition (Washington, D.C.: Department of Health and Human Services).

2. Morrison, P. "Work and Retirement in an Aging Society," *Daedelus* 115: 269–93 (1986).

3. Palmer, J. and S. Gould. "The Economic Consequences of an Aging Society," *Daedelus* 114: 295–323 (1986).

4. Under prospective payment, Medicare inpatient admissions declined both in 1984 and in 1985, as did average length of stay for Medicare patients. The rates still remain higher, however, than those for younger patients. Prospective Payment Assessment Commission, "Medicare Prospective Payment and the American Health Care System," Report to the Congress (Washington, D.C.: 1986).

5. Fuchs, V. " 'Though Much is Taken': Reflections on Aging, Health, and Medical Care," *Milbank Memorial Fund Quarterly/Health and Society* 62:143–66 (1984); Lubitz, J. and R. Prihoda, "The Use and Costs of Medicare Services in the Last Two Years of Life," *Health Care Financing Review* 5:117–31 (Spring, 1984). Lubitz and Prihoda point out that Medicare expenditures for care of the dying tend to be highest for cancer patients, and tend to decline as patients die at older ages, most likely because nursing home or home care substitute for inpatient hospital care, and because illnesses tend to lead to death more quickly. They also argue that there is no evidence that expenditures on the dying have added disproportionately to increases in Medicare expenditures during the last few years.

6. Aaron, H. and W. Schwartz. *The Painful Prescription*. Washington, D.C.: Brookings Institution (1984).

2

The Fourth Stage of the Epidemiologic Transition: The Age of Delayed Degenerative Diseases

S. Jay Olshansky

A. Brian Ault

Abstract

GAINS IN LONGEVITY in the United States since the middle of the 19th century occurred as a result of an epidemiologic transition; deaths from infectious and parasitic diseases were replaced by deaths from degenerative diseases. Generally, the consequence of this transition was a redistribution of deaths from the young to the old. The epidemiologic transition theory, as it was set forth by its originator, Abdel Omran, described the three stages of the transition as "The Age of Pestilence and Famine (lasting until about 1850), The Age of Receding Pandemics (lasting from 1850 to 1920), and the Age of Degenerative and Man-made Diseases (lasting from 1920 on)." Recent trends in cause-specific mortality indicate that since the mid-1960s in the United States there have been rapid declines in deaths from major degenerative diseases, primarily among the population reaching advanced ages. This has resulted in unexpected increases in life expect-

Funding for this research was provided by the Administration on Aging grant no. 90AL0012 through the Intermountain West Long-term Care Gerontology Center at the University of Utah, and Department of Energy contract no. W-31-109-ENG-38 at Argonne National Laboratory. This paper was previously published in *The Milbank Quarterly* vol. 64 no. 3 (1986): 355–91.

ancy at birth and at older ages that go beyond the general characteristics of what is described as the third stage of epidemiologic transition. The timing and magnitude of this latest mortality transition is significant and distinct enough from the previous three stages to qualify as the Fourth Stage of the Epidemiologic Transition—a stage characterized by the postponement of death from degenerative diseases. Observed and projected period life tables provided by the United States Office of the Actuary, and mortality counts published by the National Center for Health Statistics for selected decades in the United States are used to illustrate this fourth stage. The results are discussed with reference to policy implications associated with population aging and health care.

Introduction

Since the turn of the century to 1980, life expectancy at birth in the United States has increased from 47 to 73.6 years. To gain a perspective of the magnitude and timing of this increase, it is estimated that it took the previous 2000 years to achieve a comparable increase for the entire human species (Dublin et al. 1949). The cause of the rapid increase in life expectancy in this century is a shift to degenerative causes of death, such as heart disease and cancer, from deaths previously caused by infectious and parasitic diseases. This shift in disease patterns has been referred to as the epidemiologic transition (Omran 1971).

According to the theory of the epidemiologic transition, nations tend to improve their social, economic, and health conditions as they modernize. Conditions conducive to the spread of infectious and parasitic diseases are rapidly replaced by more sanitary living conditions, improved medical technology, and more healthful lifestyles. As the risk of dying from infectious diseases is reduced for a population, those saved from dying from such diseases survive into middle and older ages where they face the elevated risk of dying from "degenerative or man-made diseases." Since degenerative diseases tend to kill at much older ages than infectious diseases, this transition in causes of death generally is characterized by a redistribution of deaths from the young to the old.

The epidemiologic transition theory, as originally set forth, was designed to provide a general picture of the major determinants of death that prevailed during several distinct periods in our epidemiologic history. In order to set forth the general characteristics of what is described in this paper as the fourth stage of the epidemiologic transition, it is necessary to define more precisely the components that make up each stage of the transition. As a way of reconceptualizing the epidemiologic transition theory, it is appropriate to identify three basic components of epidemiologic change that distinguish one stage from another.

The first component was identified originally by Omran (1971) as shifts in recorded cause-of-death patterns. Trends in causes of death are observed most frequently as a ratio of the relative contributions of each cause of death to deaths from all causes, or more simply as changes in the relative ranking of the ten leading causes of death. Rapid changes in cause-of-death patterns imply that a major transition in the general health status of the population has taken place.

The second component involves the age and sex groups of the population that are affected by mortality transitions. The importance of following changes in patterns of death among different age and sex groups is that one may determine, first, whether some subgroups of the population are benefitting more or less than others from changes in the population's general health status, and second, it provides more detailed information on the relative risk of death by cause for population subgroups.

The third component of epidemiologic change is the effects of transitions in causes of death on survival. Here, we ask the fundamental question, "Who benefits the most from mortality transitions in terms of gains in life expectancy?" The importance of this component is that it identifies the benefactors of declining mortality not just in terms of changes in the risk of dying, but in terms of a concept that is understood more easily—the number of years of life gained. Also, by observing relative changes in longevity for different age and sex groups as a function of mortality change across the age structure, it is possible to pinpoint where the largest gains in longevity are concentrated.

If we evaluate the first stage of the epidemiologic transition (the Age of Pestilence and Famine) using these three components, we note first that this stage is characterized, not by changes in average death rates, but by a stagnation of death rates at extremely high levels for a period of what is believed to be thousands of years. During this stage, death rates fluctuated at very high levels between peaks and troughs in response to epidemics that periodically ravaged the population. The major killers during this era included influenza, pneumonia, diarrhea, smallpox, tuberculosis, and other related diseases. Infants and children died more frequently from the major killers of this era, although women of reproductive age also faced an unusually high risk of death because of the complications associated with pregnancy and delivery. Since the major causes of death during this time tended to take their greatest toll on the young, the effects on survival are profound in that the median age at death is skewed heavily toward younger ages, and life expectancy hovers somewhere between 20 and 40.

The second stage (the Age of Receding Pandemics) is transitional, and is characterized most by rapid changes in the components of our epidemiologic history. During this stage, the peaks and troughs of mortality were smoothed out initially by rapid improvements in sanitation and standards of living, with medical and public health measures contributing significantly after mid-century (McKinlay and McKinlay 1977; Chen and Wagner 1978). With health and social conditions improving, those who would have previously succumbed to infectious and parasitic diseases survive through their early years into middle and older ages where they face an elevated risk of dying from chronic degenerative diseases. Since degenerative diseases, and infectious and parasitic diseases tend to kill at opposite ends of the age structure, the transformation in causes of death during this era resulted in a redistribution of death from the young to the old. The most favorable effects on survival were, therefore, concentrated among infants, children, and women of childbearing age, which resulted in increased prospects for surviving to and through adulthood. During this stage, life expectancy at birth increased to about 50 years of age.

The third stage (the Age of Degenerative and Man-Made Diseases) has been described basically as a plateau phase in our epidemiologic history during which we again reach a level of equilibrium in mortality, but at a level considerably lower than that of the first stage. In this stage, the pace of the declines in mortality rates throughout the age structure slows as the theoretical limits to mortality declines are approached. The major causes of death for the population are chronic degenerative diseases such as heart disease, cancer, and stroke, which tend to kill at ages near what was believed to be the end of the life span. The effect on longevity is a life expectancy for the population that reaches into seven decades of life and was expected to change little in the future.

When this general theory of mortality change was published in 1971, there was reason to believe that mortality declines had bottomed out, and gains in life expectancy from that time forward would progress at a snail's pace. The rationale for that belief was that there had to be limits to declining mortality as the biological limit to life is approached, and it was generally believed, at the time, that seven decades of life was close to that limit.

A few years prior to the publication of the epidemiologic transition theory, the United States and other developed nations began to experience unexpectedly rapid declines in mortality rates for the major degenerative diseases. In the United States, for example, heart disease declined by more than 25 percent between 1968 and 1978 (U.S. Department of Health and Human Services 1981), and there is evidence to indicate that such declines have continued, and are expected to continue into the future (Gillum et al. 1984; Havlick and Feinleib 1979). Death rates for other degenerative diseases, such as cancer and stroke, have also declined since the early 1970s (U.S. Department of Health and Human Services 1980; U.S. Department of Health, Education and Welfare 1982). While the greatest benefits of these declining death rates were experienced first by the population passing through their middle ages, today, some of the largest declines are occurring among those from whom one might least expect them— cohorts recently passing through advanced ages. Furthermore, data on international trends in cause-specific mortality indicate that the majority of the declining age-specific death rates are occurring as a result of declining mortality for major cardiovascular diseases. This new trend is known to have begun in the mid-1960s (Pisa and Uemura 1985; Uemura and Pisa 1982; Rosenwaike et al. 1980). A 25 percent decline in the nation's number one cause of death within a ten-year time period is a remarkable achievement in itself, but when it occurs for a degenerative disease among the population in advanced ages, it may be considered a major achievement in our epidemiologic history.

This unanticipated decline in death rates from degenerative diseases raises two important questions. First, why did this transition begin at that particular time in our epidemiologic history—in the mid-1960s—and just after it appeared that mortality rates had reached a lower plateau? And second, what precipitated this new stage and what is currently sustaining the continuation of this phase today?

In answering these questions, it is possible to identify several historical circumstances that are generally believed to have contributed to this new era in our epidemiologic history. First, the mortality transition that occurred during "the Age of Receding Pandemics" created a fundamental change in the prospects for survival and in the age structure of the United States population. From an historical perspective, we are literally transformed overnight from a relatively young population with a broadly based age structure through the mid-19th century, into a rapidly aging population. Within just 50 years from the turn of the century, the median age of the United States population had increased from 22.9 to 30.2, and the proportion of the total population aged 65 and over had increased from 4.1 percent to 8.1 percent (U.S. Bureau of the Census 1975). This fundamental change in the age structure, with rapidly increasing proportions of successive birth cohorts surviving into advanced ages, literally created an entirely new segment of the population with unique health care needs and demands that were tied to chronic degenerative diseases and age-associated physiological impairments.

Moreover, by the second half of the 20th century, significant declines in infant and child mortality had largely been achieved for the majority of the United States population, and the health care community began to focus its attention more on the chronic degenerative conditions that plagued the survivors into advanced ages. With the development of new drugs and antibiotics and improved methods of diagnosing and treating degenerative diseases and their complications, the health care community became increasingly successful in postponing deaths from degenerative diseases by slowing the rate of chronic disease progression and by reducing case fatality rates (U.S. Department of Health and Human Services 1980; Watkins 1984; Manton 1982).

Finally, advances in medical technology were accompanied by reductions in some major risk factors for degenerative diseases (on a population scale) such as declines in smoking, more exercise, and improved dietary habits (Havlick and Feinleib 1979; Walker 1977; Watkins 1984; Gillum 1984). Moreover, federal health care programs begun in the 1960s were targeted primarily at the elderly and poor segments of the population, and are thought to have contributed to mortality declines by reducing inequities in access to quality health care.

The combination of all of these factors: improved survival and a pronounced shift in the age structure toward older ages; recent advances in medical technology and public health measures that favored the old over the young; federal health care programs that favored the elderly and poor; and reductions in risk factors on a population scale, are largely responsible for this new era in our epidemiologic history. However, the relative contributions of each of these circumstances to declining mortality has yet to be determined. In effect, prospects for improved survival were then largely concentrated among those segments of the population that were increasing the fastest, in terms of both absolute numbers and proportions— cohorts passing through advanced ages—thus leading to rapid declines in death rates from major degenerative diseases on a population scale.

As a result of this unexpected transition among degenerative diseases, the expectation of life at birth in the United States has risen rapidly in recent years to the upper end of the seventh decade of life, and among some populations in the developed world, life expectancy has already reached eight decades. It is generally recognized now that life expectancy for some developed nations will reach well into the eighth decade by the turn of the century. More interestingly, however, such gains in longevity have been, and are likely to continue to be propelled into eight decades by unprecedented and significant mortality declines among the cohorts that will reach advanced ages in the coming decades (Myers 1983).

The timing and magnitude of this mortality transition is significant and distinct enough from the previous three stages to qualify as the Fourth Stage of the Epidemiologic Transition. The general characteristics of the fourth stage include 1) rapidly declining death rates that are concentrated mostly in advanced ages and that occur at nearly the same pace for males and females, 2) the age pattern of mortality by cause remains largely the same as in the third stage, but the age distribution of deaths for degenerative causes are shifted progressively toward older ages, and 3) relatively rapid improvements in survival are concentrated among the population in advanced ages. Thus, in this stage, the major degenerative causes of death that prevailed during the third stage of the transition remain with us as the major killers, but the risk of dying from these diseases is redistributed to older ages. This unexpected shift in the age pattern of mortality for degenerative causes for the population in advanced ages is what is so unique about the fourth stage, and is its major distinguishing characteristic from the third stage of the transition. Since this stage is characterized most by a substitution of the ages at which the major determinants of death prevailing at the time tend to kill, this stage in our epidemiologic history will be referred to as "the Age of Delayed Degenerative Diseases." I will use mortality data from the United States to illustrate the timing and magnitude of this fourth stage.

The United States Experience

As a result of the epidemiologic transition, today in the United States approximately three of every four deaths occur as a result of degenerative disease, primarily in advanced ages. We have achieved such remarkable success in reducing death rates in younger and middle ages that now there is relatively little room left for improvement barring the reduction of accidents, homicide, and suicide. This means that if *significant* mortality declines and gains in life expectancy are to be achieved in the future, they will have to occur as a result of achievements made at older ages.

Recent data suggest, in fact, that older generations throughout the developed world have achieved some remarkable declines in mortality and gains in life expectancy in advanced ages (Manton 1984; Lopez and Hanada 1982). In fact, recent research on mortality patterns in advanced ages for the United States indicate that significant mortality declines are occurring in every age group beyond the age of 65 (Crimmins 1984; U.S. Department of Health and Human Services 1984). Mortality declines of this magnitude in advanced ages are considered remarkable, because it is believed that as a population we are now rapidly approaching the biological limit to life, and it takes increasingly larger investments from the health care industry to achieve even small returns as gains in life expectancy. The issue of determining the age of the biological limit to life, however, is not without debate, as we may note from recent articles on this topic (Myers and Manton 1984; Fries 1984). Moreover, it is questionable as to how long we may successfully reap longevity benefits from improving risk factors and delaying degenerative causes of death into advanced ages.

In the sections that follow, I will analyze complete life tables by decade for males and females in the United States from 1900 to 1980, and projected complete life tables to the year 2020. The life tables were published by the United States Office of the Actuary (Faber 1982). Mortality projections were performed by analyzing average annual improvements in central death rates by age, sex, and ten leading causes of death for the period 1968 to 1978, and extrapolating these trends forward in time based upon assumptions of how such factors as advance in research, environmental pollution, incidence of violence, continued improvements in lifestyles, and personal responsibility for health care might influence mortality. Mortality counts published by the National Center for Health Statistics (1963, 1974, 1985) are also used in this analysis.

The timing and magnitude of the fourth stage of the epidemiologic transition will be illustrated by examining trends in life expectancy, temporary life expectancies, survival curves, a decomposition of changes in temporary life expectancies into the relative contributions of mortality change made by selected age ranges, and recent shifts in the age distributions of death for selected degenerative diseases.

Life Expectancy

Table 2.1 shows life expectancy at selected ages for the United States observed from 1900 to 1980, and projected to the year 2020 based upon estimates made by the United States Office of the Actuary. Two notable patterns emerge. First, in the early part of this century, the largest absolute and percentage increases in life expectancy occurred in younger age groups. For example, from 1900 to 1920, females gained 7.3 years (14.8%) at birth and only .13 years (3.3%) at age 85. By the end of this century, the United States Office of the Actuary projects a slowdown in gains in life expectancy at birth and relatively

Table 2.1 Observed (1900–1980) and Projected (1990–2020) Life Expectancy at Selected Exact Ages in the Unites States, by Sex*

Ages	1900 (1)	1910 (2)	1920 (3)	1930 (4)	1940 (5)	1950 (6)	1960 (7)	1970 (8)	1980 (9)	1990 (10)	2000 (11)	2010 (12)	2020 (13)
Males													
0	46.56	50.20	54.59	58.01	60.89	65.33	66.58	67.05	69.85	72.29	73.42	73.93	74.42
20	41.73	42.63	44.45	45.14	46.77	49.01	49.65	49.64	51.64	53.71	54.76	55.23	55.68
40	27.52	27.64	29.20	28.82	29.42	30.87	31.32	31.56	33.42	35.26	36.20	36.67	37.12
60	14.18	14.18	14.87	14.69	14.84	15.75	15.86	16.11	17.29	18.55	19.24	19.64	20.03
85	3.73	3.88	3.95	4.12	4.05	4.49	4.61	4.74	5.08	5.63	6.00	6.23	6.47
Females													
0	49.07	53.67	56.33	61.36	65.34	70.90	73.19	74.80	77.53	79.85	81.05	81.62	82.18
20	42.90	44.98	44.83	47.51	50.24	53.86	55.62	56.82	58.90	60.94	62.06	62.60	63.13
40	28.69	29.57	30.06	31.01	32.54	35.19	36.64	37.87	39.69	41.58	42.65	43.18	43.70
60	14.96	15.16	15.48	16.04	16.78	18.61	19.57	20.88	22.20	23.79	24.70	25.19	25.66
85	4.00	4.06	4.13	4.41	4.36	4.98	5.11	5.72	6.32	7.23	7.82	8.13	8.44

*Source: Faber, J. 1982. Life Tables for the United States: 1900–2050. Social Security Administration. SSA Pub. No. 11-11534.

rapid gains in longevity in advanced ages. Over the 40-year time period from the year 1980 to 2020, for instance, absolute and percentage increases in life expectancy for females are projected to be 2.12 years (33.5%) at age 85, and 4.65 years (6.0%) at age zero, respectively. Similar patterns are projected for males. This represents a complete reversal of trends in mortality and life expectancy where gains that previously occurred in younger ages are now replaced by relatively large increases in life expectancy in advanced ages.

Also, sex differences in life expectancy at birth have increased steadily from 1900 until the decade of the '70s (except for a brief time period during the influenza epidemic in 1918). They are then projected to decrease by 1990 and then increase to the difference that was observed in 1970. Although explanations for these sex differences in life expectancy are complex, it is important to note that the historical pattern of a widening gap in longevity between the sexes is projected to come to an end during the fourth stage of the epidemiologic transition in the United States. Whether this trend will hold true for other developed nations has yet to be determined.

Temporary Life Expectancies

Table 2.2 shows observed and projected changes in temporary life expectancies at selected ages for males and females. A temporary life expectancy (TLE) may be interpreted as the average number of years that a group of persons at exact age x will live from age x to $x + i$. The temporary life expectancy from birth to age 85, for example, is considered a more reliable measure of changes in life expectancy at birth than using e_x^o because it avoids problems of data reliability at older ages. The calculation of the TLEs also provide an estimate of the relative changes occurring in life expectancy within selected age ranges that occur as a result of mortality changes in age groups within those age ranges (Arriaga 1984).

For example, a figure of 46.38 for males in 1900 at age interval "birth to age 85" means that for male babies born in 1900, they could expect to live an average of 46.38 years if they experienced the mortality rates of the period in which they were born, throughout their lives. The figure of 24.76 for females in 1980 at age interval 20–45 means that for those who reached their twentieth birthday in 1980, they could expect to live an average of 24.76 out of a possible 25 years in the age interval. If the TLE for the age interval was 25, then virtually everyone who reached their twentieth birthday would also be assured of reaching their forty-fifth birthday (i.e, zero deaths in the age interval).

According to these data, TLEs increased rapidly throughout this

Table 2.2 Observed (1900–1980) and Projected (1990–2020) Changes in Temporary Life Expectancies at Selected Exact Age Intervals for the United States, by Sex*

Ages	1900 (1)	1910 (2)	1920 (3)	1930 (4)	1940 (5)	1950 (6)	1960 (7)	1970 (8)	1980 (9)	Projected 1990 (10)	2000 (11)	2010 (12)	2020 (13)
Birth to Age 85													
Males	46.38	50.00	54.32	57.70	60.55	64.80	66.00	66.41	68.96	71.02	71.91	72.27	72.60
Females	48.82	53.37	55.99	60.88	64.75	69.85	71.92	73.05	75.15	76.58	77.22	77.50	77.76
Birth to Age 20													
Males	15.62	16.48	17.39	18.13	18.45	19.08	19.24	19.40	19.62	19.71	19.73	19.75	19.76
Females	16.15	16.95	17.80	18.47	18.78	19.29	19.43	19.54	19.71	19.78	19.80	19.81	19.82
Ages 20–45													
Males	22.62	22.95	23.14	23.54	23.97	24.29	24.37	24.28	24.35	24.46	24.50	24.51	24.52
Females	22.69	23.21	22.98	23.68	24.18	24.56	24.67	24.67	24.76	24.81	24.82	24.83	24.83
Ages 45–65													
Males	16.80	16.85	17.32	17.15	17.32	17.64	17.77	17.82	18.23	18.55	18.69	18.74	18.78
Females	17.09	17.41	17.52	17.70	18.10	18.54	18.78	18.82	19.04	19.19	19.26	19.29	19.32
Ages 65–85													
Males	10.87	10.88	11.25	11.22	11.31	11.94	12.00	12.14	12.76	13.42	13.76	13.95	14.14
Females	11.41	11.47	11.67	12.07	12.52	13.65	14.26	14.92	15.50	16.11	16.40	16.55	16.69

Source: Calculated from data published by Faber (1982).

century in all age groups and for almost all time periods (excluding 1920–1930 for males aged 45 and older, females aged 20–45 from 1910–1920, and males aged 20–45 from 1960–1970). The largest absolute increases within age ranges occurred in the earlier part of this century with smaller increases projected to occur by the year 2020. Note that in the two youngest age intervals (0–20 and 20–45) during this century, the TLEs rapidly approach the size of the age interval, thus indicating that mortality is already so low in these age ranges that further improvements will be difficult to achieve. For this reason, the magnitude of the increases in TLEs is projected to decrease past 1990, except in the oldest age interval where there is still room and expectation for further improvements.

Basically, these data provide a clear picture of the magnitude of the potential gains in longevity that remain for the different age-sex groups in the United States. Females in 1980, for example, had less than one-third and one-quarter of a year of life that remained to be achieved within the two younger age intervals, respectively. In the oldest age group in 1980, about 4.5 years remained to be achieved for females. Projections to the year 2020 indicate that the oldest age groups for both males and females will achieve the largest relative increases in TLEs. This illustrates the point that if life expectancy at birth increases in the future, it will have to occur primarily as a result of mortality declines in the age groups where there is still room for improvement—older cohorts.

Index of Annual Relative Change

While TLEs are useful, they do not provide one with a true picture of the *pace* of the relative gains in longevity over time because absolute gains should be considered in relation to the maximum possible change that may occur (Arriaga 1984). For example, the projected 4.57 and 4.65 year increase in life expectancy at birth for males and females, respectively, from 1980 to 2020 may be interpreted as a 6.5 percent increase for males and a 6 percent increase for females. One might conclude from this that males are expected to make the greater achievement of the two sexes by the year 2020. However, when these projected gains in life expectancy at birth are shown as a proportion of the maximum possible change (let us say the difference between the observed life expectancy and a biological limit to life estimated at 100 years of age), then males would experience a 15.2 percent increase toward the biological limit to life while females would experience a 20.7 percent increase toward the same biological limit to life (using the age of 100 as an illustration of the biological limit to life for males and females). Under this interpretation, the greater achievement is now thought to go to females. The same logic may be applied when calculating observed and projected gains in TLEs within selected age ranges. One way to address this issue of relative change in life expectancy is to calculate an index of annual relative change.

Table 2.3 shows observed and projected indices of annual relative change in selected TLEs for the United States for decades from 1900 to 2020. This measure may be interpreted as the annual percentage change in life expectancy within a given age range as a proportion of the maximum possible change. For example, the figure of 3.13 for females in 1970–1980 in the age range 20–45 may be interpreted as an annual 3.13 percent increase toward the maximum possible change in the TLE during that decade.

The data in Table 2.3 suggest that, while there were some rather dramatic fluctuations in the pace of improvements in TLEs, for the most part, the largest gains occurred between 1930 and 1950 across the age structure. The pace of the improvements then declined until 1970 during which they again increased unexpectedly for most age-sex groups. This corresponds with the onset of rapid declines in coronary heart disease mortality and other degenerative causes of death. This general pattern of fluctuations held true in all age ranges except the oldest, where the pace of relative improvements peaked in the decade of the '40s, declined in the decade of the '50s, and then gradually increased again to a peak projected for the decade of the '80s. Past 1990, the pace of improvements in TLEs in all age ranges was projected to taper off rapidly. In effect, this means that for those who reached the beginning of each age interval during these years, successively larger proportions have been observed to survive, and are projected to survive, to the subsequent age interval. This rapid decline in the pace of improvements in TLEs is expected since the data in Table 2.2 suggest that the TLEs in the younger age groups have rapidly approached the size of the age interval and the limits to further declines.

Survival Curves

A changing pattern of survival during this century among younger vs. older cohorts may be observed from the survival curves in Figures 2.1 and 2.2. Note that in 1900 there were rapid declines in the survival curves in the first few years of life with rapidly declining infant and child mortality. As the diseases that affect the young were replaced by degenerative diseases, more people survived through their first few years of life into middle and older ages, which subsequently led to a much slower drop-off of the survival curve for both sexes (shown here for 1940 and 1980). Projections of survival to the year 2020

Table 2.3 Observed (1900–1980) and Projected (1990–2020) Index of Annual Relative Change in Selected Exact Temporary Life Expectancies in the United States, by Sex*

Ages	1900/ 1910 (1)	1910/ 1920 (2)	1920/ 1930 (3)	1930/ 1940 (4)	1940/ 1950 (5)	1950/ 1960 (6)	1960/ 1970 (7)	1970/ 1980 (8)	Projected 1980/ 1990 (9)	1990/ 2000 (10)	2000/ 2010 (11)	2010/ 2020 (12)
Birth to Age 85												
Males	0.98	1.31	1.16	1.10	1.89	0.61	0.22	1.46	1.37	0.66	0.28	0.26
Females	1.34	0.86	1.83	1.73	2.86	1.46	0.90	1.91	1.56	0.79	0.37	0.35
Birth to Age 20												
Males	2.16	2.95	3.28	1.86	5.08	1.89	2.34	4.46	2.67	0.71	0.77	0.41
Females	2.30	3.21	3.57	2.24	5.27	2.17	2.12	4.51	2.72	0.95	0.51	0.54
Ages 20–45												
Males	1.48	0.97	2.39	3.43	3.65	1.19	−1.34	1.02	1.84	0.77	0.20	0.21
Females	2.52	−1.22	4.17	4.65	6.04	2.84	0.00	3.13	2.31	0.54	0.57	0.00
Ages 45–65												
Males	0.16	1.60	−0.62	0.61	1.26	0.57	0.23	2.06	1.97	1.01	0.39	0.32
Females	1.16	0.43	0.75	1.89	2.60	1.78	0.33	2.04	1.68	0.90	0.41	0.43
Ages 65–85												
Males	0.01	0.41	−0.03	0.10	0.75	0.07	0.18	0.82	0.95	0.53	0.31	0.32
Females	0.07	0.24	0.49	0.58	1.62	1.00	1.21	1.21	1.45	0.77	0.42	0.41

Source: Calculated from data published by Faber (1982).

illustrate that older generations will gain significantly more than any other part of the age structure. This may be observed by noting that the vertical increase in the survival curve is greater in older ages than in younger ages between 1980 and 2020. Also, observe how the median age at death is being pushed farther in the direction of older ages so that by the year 2020 half of the birth cohorts for those years are projected to survive to ages 77 and 86, respectively, for males and females (see Table 2.4). In fact, more than eight of every ten people born in the year 2020 are projected to survive to their eighty-fifth birthday. Since relatively small gains in survival are projected to occur for younger and middle age groups in the coming decades, this shift in the median age at death must necessarily be effected by declining mortality in advanced ages. This is a complete reversal of the patterns of improved survival that occurred earlier in this century.

Contributions to Gains in Longevity

To best illustrate the recent gains in mortality in advanced ages and the importance of such gains to changes in life expectancy, we should examine the relative contributions to gains in longevity that are made by observed and projected mortality change within selected age ranges. This will serve to illustrate *shifts* in the relative importance of different age groups to observed and projected gains in TLEs during this century.

Table 2.5 illustrates how mortality patterns during this century have contributed to patterns of change in the TLE from birth to age 85 from 1900 to 1980, and the extent of its contribution in the future

---

Table 2.4   Median Age at Death and Proportion Surviving to Ages 65 and 85, by Sex (United States, 1900-2020)

Sex	1900 (1)	1940 (2)	1980 (3)	2020 (4)
	Median Age at Death (in years)			
Males	55	67	73	77
Females	58	72	81	86
	Proportion Surviving to Age 65			
Males	37.4	55.0	70.3	78.6
Females	41.1	65.0	83.5	87.8
	Proportion Surviving to Age 85			
Males	4.7	8.2	17.5	28.1
Females	6.2	13.4	37.6	52.4

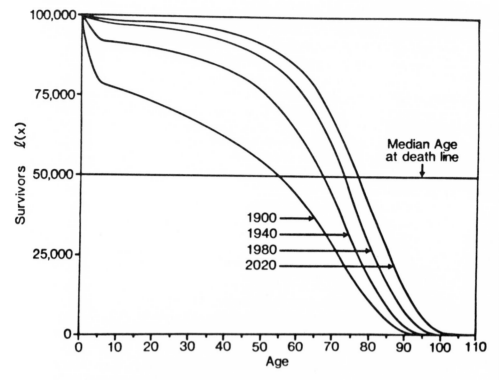

Figure 2.1 Survival curves for U.S. males (1900–2020)

based upon United States Office of the Actuary projections. According to these data, in the first two decades of this century, the mortality change in the youngest age interval (0–20) contributed from two-thirds to over three-quarters of the gains in the TLE from birth to age 85 in those decades. For example, of the 3.62 year gain in the TLE for males from 1900 to 1910, 82 percent or 2.97 of those years gained were caused by mortality declines among the population ages 0–20. Less than four percent of the increase was attributable to mortality change from the oldest age interval (65–85) for either sex during these decades. This finding is consistent with the transformation in patterns of diseases that occurred during the second stage of the epidemiologic transition.

The substitution of degenerative diseases for infectious diseases leads to rapid mortality declines in younger ages, since it is these age groups that face the highest risk of dying from infectious diseases. During this century, we may observe that with each succeeding decade the contributions to gains in TLEs from the youngest age groups are replaced by greater contributions made by older age

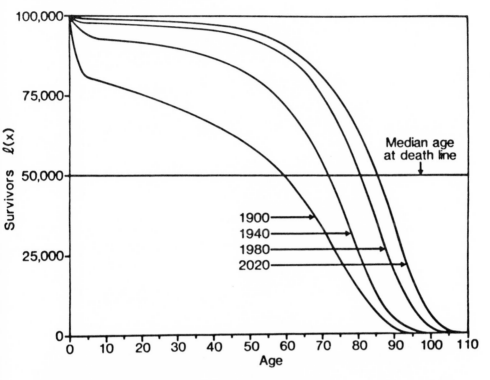

Figure 2.2 Survival curves for U.S. females (1900–2020)

groups. Negative values indicate that mortality actually increased during the decade for that age group and, thus, had a competing and negative effect on the observed change in the TLE. This explains the rather inconsistently smaller increases in the TLEs for females in the decade 1910–1920, and for males in the decade 1960–1970, in light of otherwise large gains in TLEs in previous and existing decades for other population subgroups. By the turn of the twenty-first century, the oldest age groups are projected to contribute significantly larger proportions to gains in life expectancy by comparison with younger age groups.

Within specific age groups, the United States Office of the Actuary has projected different patterns of change. For example, for both sexes, the relative contributions to gains in longevity from the youngest age group (0–20) are projected to level off by 1990 at approximately 15 percent of the contribution to changes in TLEs from birth to age 85. The second age interval (20–45) is projected to make successively smaller contributions since mortality in these ages has already declined to such low levels that further significant declines are not

Table 2.5 Observed (1900-1980) and Projected (1980—2020) Contribution of the Mortality Changes in Selected Exact Age Groups to the Total Change in Temporary Life Expectancy from Birth to Age 85 in the United States, by Sex

Ages	1900/ 1910 (1)	1910/ 1920 (2)	1920/ 1930 (3)	1930/ 1940 (4)	1940/ 1950 (5)	1950/ 1960 (6)	1960/ 1970 (7)	1970/ 1980 (8)	Projected 1980/ 1990 (9)	Projected 1990/ 2000 (10)	Projected 2000/ 2010 (11)	Projected 2010/ 2020 (12)
Males												
TLE Increase (in years)	(3.62)	(4.32)	(3.38)	(2.85)	(4.25)	(1.20)	(0.41)	(2.55)	(2.06)	(0.89)	(0.36)	(0.33)
0–20	82.0	74.7	83.5	50.3	56.3	52.7	114.7	33.5	20.4	11.7	15.4	12.5
20–45	16.7	4.9	25.4	39.6	23.1	24.7	–60.0	14.6	19.7	20.0	9.6	8.8
45–65	1.2	16.5	–8.5	8.5	12.5	19.5	24.6	36.2	37.3	39.6	35.4	34.4
65–85	0.1	3.9	–0.4	1.6	8.1	3.1	20.7	15.7	22.6	28.7	39.6	44.3
All Ages	100.0	100.0	100.0	100.0	100.0	100.0	100.0	100.0	100.0	100.0	100.0	100.0
Females												
TLE Increase (in years)	(4.55)	(2.62)	(4.89)	(3.87)	(5.10)	(2.07)	(1.13)	(2.10)	(1.43)	(0.64)	(0.28)	(0.26)
0–20	65.8	105.4	55.5	38.5	42.7	29.0	37.7	32.7	26.6	14.0	14.7	15.1
20–45	25.1	–16.4	35.0	36.0	24.4	20.9	0.7	19.2	15.4	15.0	9.0	5.4
45–65	8.6	7.3	5.4	18.8	18.5	28.2	15.7	26.2	24.9	31.0	31.4	33.2
65–85	0.5	3.7	4.1	6.7	14.4	21.9	45.9	21.9	33.1	40.0	44.9	46.3
All Ages	100.0	100.0	100.0	100.0	100.0	100.0	100.0	100.0	100.0	100.0	100.0	100.0

expected. Contributions previously made by younger age groups are projected to be replaced by contributions to gains in TLEs made by older age groups, with the largest contribution projected to be made by the population aged 65–85.

It should be noted, however, that the increased relative contributions to gains in TLEs by older cohorts will occur under conditions where the absolute TLE increases are projected to be much smaller than that experienced in previous decades. The timing of this decrease and the pace of improving TLEs shown here is a function of the assumption about mortality change made by the United States Office of the Actuary. Such a decline is expected to occur as we approach the biological limits to mortality declines, although the time period in which mortality compression will occur is still in question. Nevertheless, this transformation in the relative importance of mortality change at opposite ends of the age structure during this century illustrates clearly another dimension of the movement into the fourth stage of the epidemiologic transition.

Shifts in the Age Distribution of Death

Although the first three stages of the epidemiologic transition have been characterized by a substitution of one set of diseases for another, it is implied here that the fourth stage is characterized by a substitution of the *ages* at which degenerative diseases tend to kill. In effect, this means that, while it is likely that degenerative diseases will remain with us as major causes of death, the risk of dying from these diseases during this stage in our transition is thought to be progressively redistributed from younger to older ages.

Evidence for this redistribution process exists in the literature. For example, Manton (1984) analyzed the distribution of the age at death for the United States population from 1962 to 1979. It was determined that for all causes the mean age at death had increased by 3.2 years for males and 5.8 years for females from 1962 to 1979. Increases in the mean age at death imply that for these selected time periods the distribution of death for the population was shifting in the direction of older ages. Similar shifts had also occurred for the population aged 60 and over, and for specific major degenerative causes of death. Interestingly, the standard deviations of ages at death had also increased during this time period for the population aged 60 and over. This implies that instead of a compression of mortality in advanced ages that has been hypothesized by other researchers (Fries 1980; Fries and Crapo 1981), there is some dispersion in the distribution of death occurring in conjunction with the delays. This shift in the distribution of death, however, cannot go on indefinitely in the face of a biological limit to life, and it is therefore inevitable that mortality compression will eventually occur.

Manton (1984) has illustrated this delay process using means and standard deviations of ages at death. Another way of following this delay process is to observe changes in the percentage distribution of deaths through the age structure for all causes and specified degenerative causes of death. If a shift in the age progression of mortality is occurring, then we would expect that for successive time periods there would be relatively fewer deaths in younger ages and increases in the percentage distribution of deaths in older ages. This is the equivalent of simply shifting the age distribution of deaths for a given year a selected number of years along the x-axis in the direction of older ages while leaving constant the relationship of the curves to one another. With a shift *and* a compression of mortality, we would expect the distribution to appear more narrow and show a higher peak in older ages by comparison to previous years.

In Figure 2.3, we see the percentage distribution of all causes of death for males and females to ages 40 and over in the United States for the decades 1960 through 1980. According to this figure, in each succeeding decade, a consistent pattern emerged where deaths that previously had occurred in younger ages were replaced by a larger proportion of deaths in advanced ages. Note how the peak ages of death occurred 10 years later and were less dispersed for females (75–89) than for males (65–79). Within sex groups from 1960 to 1980, it appears that the distribution merely shifted toward older ages with no evidence of compression.

While similar patterns emerge for the specific causes of death taken separately, there are notable exceptions. For example, while the distribution of death for ischemic heart disease (Figure 2.4) illustrates a consistent shift in the direction of older ages for successive decades for males and females, the relative distributions of death in the three peak age groups in 1980 represented 8.3 percent more of the deaths for females (52.6) than it represented for males (44.3). As a result, there was less dispersion of deaths for females. With cerebrovascular diseases, the age distributions were shifted five years farther in the direction of older ages than that which was experienced for all causes for both males and females (see Figure 2.5). In the case of malignant neoplasms (Figure 2.6), the distribution of deaths for males and females peaked at the same ages (65-74), and were relatively higher and less dispersed for males—a pattern quite different than for other degenerative causes of death.

These data suggest that while varying patterns exist in the age distribution of death by sex and for specific causes taken separately, generally, the trend from 1960 to 1980 has been toward a shift in the

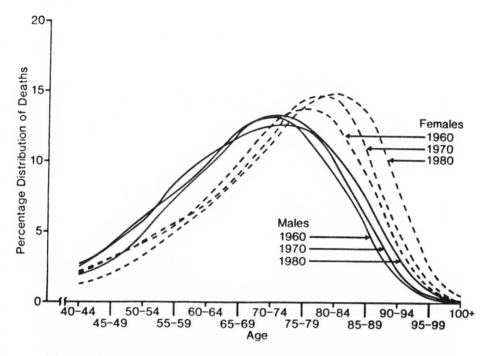

Figure 2.3 Percentage distribution of deaths from all causes for the U.S. population at ages 40 and over, by sex (1960, 1970,1980).

distribution in the direction of older ages with larger shifts occurring in the latter decade. There is also no evidence from these data on selected degenerative causes to suggest that mortality was compressed into advanced ages during the time periods considered here.

Implications

The era of delayed degenerative diseases is likely to have numerous impacts on two major demographic variables: the size and relative proportions of the population in advanced ages, and the health and vitality of the elderly.

Several studies have estimated prospective changes in the size and relative distributions of the population in advanced ages for the United States and other developed nations (Siegel 1979; Siegel 1980; Siegel and Hoover 1984; Rice and Feldman 1983). For example, Siegel (1979) has projected that by the year 2020 the population aged 65 and over in the United States will double from 23 million in 1976 to about 45 million. All segments of the elderly population are expected to grow dramatically, particularly the extreme aged (aged 85 and over). While projections of absolute numbers of the elderly are fairly reliable

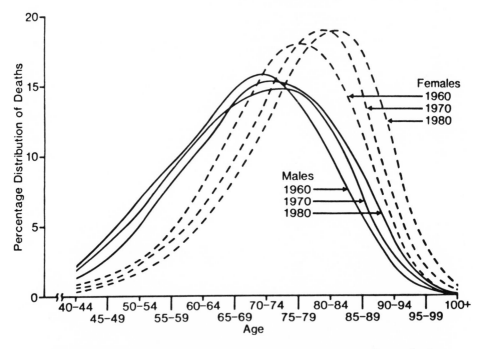

Figure 2.4 Percentage distribution of deaths from ischemic heart disease for the U.S. population at ages 40 and over, by sex (1960, 1970, 1980).

because they depend solely upon assumptions about mortality for a population that is already alive, alternative mortality assumptions based upon *delays* in degenerative diseases (instead of an extrapolation of past trends) indicate that there could be as many as 1.5 million more people over the age of 65 in the United States by the year 2020 than that projected by the United States Bureau of the Census (Olshansky 1984). In this regard, it is important to recognize that even minor differences in projection assumptions about mortality can produce rather large differences in the absolute number of people expected to be alive in advanced ages in the future.

The proportions of the elderly as a function of the total population are also expected to increase by the second decade of the next century. While the major demographic component that will bring forth increases in the absolute number and proportions of people in advanced ages is different size cohorts moving through the age structure, rapid mortality declines in advanced ages tend to accelerate the aging of the population by allowing larger proportions of successive birth cohorts to survive into advanced ages. The fourth stage of the epidemiologic transition will therefore accelerate the growth rate of the absolute numbers of elderly in the population, and it will place

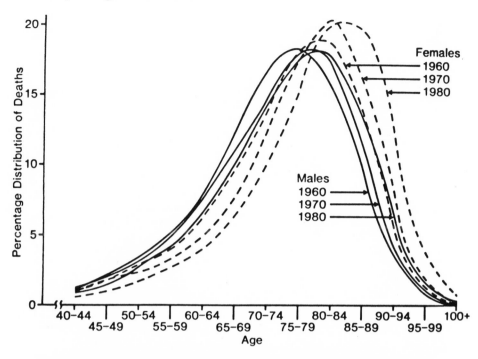

Figure 2.5 Percentage distribution of deaths from cerebrovascular disease for the U.S. population at ages 40 and over, by sex (1960, 1970, 1980).

an additional upward pressure on the rate of population aging beyond that expected from the temporal shifts in the age structure. This phenomenon of population aging is a demographic process currently being experienced by developed and developing nations throughout the world (Myers 1982).

Although the numbers and proportions of the elderly are viewed as a potential problem for social service programs, this issue is now giving ground in importance to the potential impact of declining mortality in advanced ages to issues of health care (Manton and Soldo 1985; Manton 1982). The central issue here is that of "vitality"—or the question of whether declining mortality in advanced ages will result in additional years of health or additional years of senescence. At one extreme, it has been suggested that future mortality declines will result in a simultaneous compression of mortality *and* morbidity into advanced ages (Fries 1980). At the other extreme, it has been argued that the survivors—the population "saved" as a result of declining mortality in advanced ages—may increase both the individual and aggregate number of years spend in a state of frail health or senescence by the elderly (Gruenberg 1977; Kramer 1980; Schneider and Brody 1983). It has even been suggested that both phenomenon will

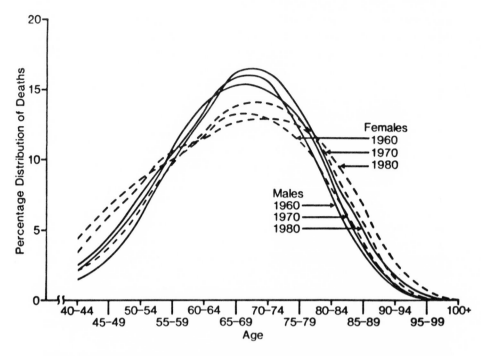

Figure 2.6 Percentage distribution of deaths from malignant neoplasms for the U.S. population at ages 40 and over, by sex (1960, 1970, 1980).

occur at the same time (Feldman 1983). That is, improved survival may lead to an increase in the proportions of the population with a short duration of functional impairment, and an increase in the proportion of the population with a longer duration of functional impairment (survivors to advanced ages in the future may experience the extremes of frailty depending upon what causes the mortality declines).

There are two other issues to consider when the topic of prospective trends in morbidity is discussed. The first involves basic demographic arithmetic. The prevalence of morbidity in a population is a product of the incidence rate and the size and age distribution of the population. Given that incidence rates of morbidity are known generally to increase as a function of age, then, as a *population* ages, there will inevitably be an accompanying increase in the prevalence of morbidity—assuming the rate of its occurrence remains constant. For example, scientists have suggested that even with declines in morbidity rates, the absolute number of people expected to reach advanced age in the near future will be so large that the effects of age composition outweigh any likely declines in the rate of morbidity, thus resulting in increased prevalence (Kramer 1980; Gruenberg 1977). Others have argued that, even with rapid increases in the absolute size of the elderly population, it is possible that the mortality declines expected to occur among cohorts reaching older ages in the future may be accompanied by a corresponding decline in the severity or rate of progression of chronic diseases, thus leading to a reduction in the incidence rate of morbidity (Manton 1982; Fries and Crapo 1981; Soldo and Manton 1985). In any case, if morbidity rates were to remain constant, then the fourth stage of the epidemiologic transition would inevitably exert an upward force on the *prevalence of morbidity*. The question is, is it reasonable to expect morbidity rates to remain constant in the face of rapid declines in death rates from major degenerative diseases?

A second issue involves the concepts of "competing causes" and "natural death." Competing causes is a term used to describe how diseases operate independently as risk factors in competition for the lives of individuals. Each cause of death is considered an independent increment to the force of mortality, and changes in the risk of dying from any single cause is thought not to influence the risk of dying from other causes. While the concept of competing causes has been used often as a method of estimating the effects on longevity of hypothetically eliminating causes of death, it is relevant to issues of morbidity-mortality linkages in that it illustrates how altering patterns of cause-specific mortality can influence a population's disease profile. Specifically, we know that if deaths for a given cause decline, then at some point in time and at some ages, the risk of dying from other causes must therefore increase. With the postponement of deaths from degenerative causes, we face the prospect of substituting, for causes of death experiencing declines, other causes of death with patterns of predeath frailty that may be significantly different than those that prevail today. For example, it is possible that with rapid declines in heart disease and cancer, there may be an increased risk of frailty from more debilitating chronic conditions such a stroke or Alzheimer's disease, or from nonlethal conditions such as arthritis and blindness (Feldman 1983). This could occur during the interim of time in which deaths from degenerative diseases are postponed, but not sufficiently so to place the survivors at an elevated risk of dying from biological constraints. Alternatively, it has been suggested that with the postponement of death from degenerative diseases, the "survivors" may live into more advanced ages and face a significantly higher risk of dying a nondisease-related "natural death," with comparatively less frailty time (Fries 1980).

The term "natural death" was introduced by Fries (1980) as a concept that represents death at the biological limit to life caused by the incremental age-associated loss of organ reserve. Fries suggested that natural death (generally acknowledged to be a condition that few people today survive long enough to experience) is the result of the natural physiologically and biologically determined process of aging that all living organisms experience, and that should be distinguished as a process separate from the age progression of chronic degenerative diseases. When the postponement of death occurs, it is suggested that the clinical manifestations of diseases are also delayed and the time available for frailty is lessened as we approach the biological limit to life (which Fries has estimated at approximately 85 years of age). However, the differences between death from biological causes and death from chronic degenerative causes are arbitrary at best. In fact, given the unrealistic assumption under competing causes that degenerative diseases operate independently of one another, it would also appear that the factors that cause "natural death" are impossibly intertwined with the factors that cause deaths from chronic degenerative diseases.

At issue here are three major assumptions relevant to estimates of morbidity. First, the nature and location of the biological limit to life is currently an issue for debate. Fries (1980) has estimated the average biological limit at about age 85, while others have estimated the biological limit at approximately 100 years of age (Cutler 1975; Havighurst and Sacher 1977). The relevance of the age of an upper bound on the life span to issues of morbidity is that this will determine the extent to which mortality will have to decline before a significant proportion of the population survive into the ages where they face an elevated risk of dying from single or multiple organ failure (if natural death is an appropriate description of death from biological causes).

It has also been suggested that the human life span may not be fixed at a single or average age at all, but instead it may actually be increasing (Manton 1982). This conclusion is based upon evidence indicating that in the United States there have been significant mortality declines among a subgroup of the population that already has the lowest mortality—white females. Perhaps, instead of a compression of mortality and morbidity against a theoretical upper limit to life, both are merely being postponed equally into later ages— leaving constant the number of years between first permanent infirmity and death. This could change the disease profile of the population, and perhaps even the duration and nature of the frailty experienced during that interval. At this time, however, it is too early to tell whether or not the life span is increasing, particularly when we consider the problems of data reliability at older ages and the unique time period we appear to have entered in our epidemiologic history.

The second assumption at issue is whether or not it is appropriate to presume that the postponement of death will be accompanied by the postponement of first permanent infirmity. Previous research (Wiley and Camacho 1980) has suggested that when mortality declines are a result of preventive health care measures, morbidity may also be postponed into later ages. However, it is not certain, first, whether this phenomenon is actually occurring and whether it will continue into the future, and second, it has yet to be determined what proportion of the mortality declines are attributable solely to preventive health care measures.

And finally, is it appropriate to assume that a biological mechanism that controls the rate of aging is separate from the age progression of chronic degenerative diseases, as Fries (1980) assumes (for more on this issue see Minaker and Rowe 1985)? Is it possible, for example, that the acquisition of healthier lifestyles on a population scale will postpone the clinical manifestations of chronic diseases and *simultaneously* slow the process of aging—thus leading to a real increase in the life span as has already been suggested (Manton 1982)? Or is it possible that the repeated insults to the body that lead to clinical manifestations of disease also accelerate the drain on organ reserve and operate to pull the biological life span (of individuals) toward younger ages? In this regard, Hayflick (1982, p. 225) has suggested that "although age-associated physiologic decrements surely increase vulnerability to disease, the fundamental causes of death are not diseases but the physiological decrements that make their occurrence more likely."

At present, the scientific evidence regarding recent patterns of morbidity in the United States is far from conclusive regarding our direction. Recent research by Verbrugge (1984), for example, indicates that the health status of the elderly population in the United States has worsened in recent decades. Feldman (1983) has shown that disability rates due to heart disease and arthritis had actually increased monotonically from 1969 to 1980 for the population aged 50–69. And McKinlay et al. (1983) have demonstrated that almost all of the increase in life expectancy that occurred in the United States from 1964 to 1974 for the cohorts reaching age 45 were disability years. Yet, for the cohorts reaching age 65 in those years, there appears to have been slight gains in the number of years free of disability. Moreover, research by Palmore (1986) indicates that the health of the population aged 65 and over in the United States may have improved from 1961 to 1981 relative to the rest of the population. In short, there is contradictory evidence regarding the issue of recent patterns of change in morbidity in the United States, and it is acknowledged that it will continue to be difficult gauging patterns of morbidity in the future because of the inherent problems associated with its measurement.

There is one final point worth mentioning with regard to the data presented here. At present, indices of mortality change indicate clearly that we have entered a new era in our epidemiologic history in terms of survival. What is most apparent from this new transition is the force it will exert toward increasing the numbers and proportions of the elderly in the population in the coming decades. Manton and Soldo (1985) have referred to a continued emphasis on the numerical aspects of aging as solely a quantitative approach to what is really a multifaceted issue—an issue that is likely to have rather unique qualitative features. For example, because of the likelihood of a finite life span and the potential for changes in the disease profile of the population, this new era in our epidemiologic history may have profound influences on basic activities of daily living for the elderly, the demands for and costs of health care services and nursing home care, health care rationing, and the case mix of elderly patients in long-term and acute care facilities. While these issues, as they relate to increased longevity and declining mortality, have been discussed extensively in the literature (Manton and Soldo 1985; Soldo and Manton 1985; Minaker and Rowe 1985; Cameron 1985; Rice and Feldman 1983; McCall 1984), a few brief points are worth mentioning here.

First, on the quantitative side, it has already been demonstrated (Rice and Feldman 1983) that projected changes in age composition alone (using the same mortality projection assumptions as in this study) will contribute significantly to a rapid growth in the demand for, and costs of, health care services (assuming there are no radical changes in age-specific morbidity rates). For example, 6 percent of the one-half billion increase in the number of annual physician visits, and more than half of the 100 percent increase in the total annual short stay hospital days that are projected to occur from 1980 to 2040, will be attributable to population aging. Furthermore, changes in age composition by the year 2040 are projected to account for a 350 percent increase in the total number of nursing home residents, a 500 percent increase in the number of nursing home residents aged 85 and over, and a $103 billion increase in the health care budget for the population aged 65 and over—assuming constant 1980 dollars. Some of the largest cost increases are projected to occur for nursing home care. It should be noted, however, that the proportional contributions of projected changes in births, deaths, migration, and age composition on the growth of the elderly population have yet to be determined.

Since the fourth stage of the epidemiologic transition will serve to allow larger proportions of successive birth cohorts to survive into advanced ages, the mortality declines projected to occur during the time frame considered here certainly will exert an additional upward pressure on health care costs and demands that go beyond that expected from different sized cohorts moving through the age structure. The nature and duration of this additional force on population aging will depend upon assumptions of how long we can expect to experience this new era in our epidemiologic history. While we know that this fourth stage must eventually come to an end, given the likelihood of a finite life span, at present there is no indication that the pace of mortality declines in advanced ages have tapered off. In fact, the mortality projection assumptions made by the United States Office of the Actuary (Faber 1982) assume a .6 percent average annual decline in mortality rates from 1981 to 2056. This is an assumption as reasonable as any other, but it should be emphasized that even small differences in mortality projection assumptions can produce significant differences in estimates of the growth of the elderly population.

It is the potential qualitative aspects of this new era, however, that force us to consider implications for other health care issues. For example, long-term care facilities and acute care settings generally treat a variety of patients that require certain kinds of care and resource requirements. The consumption of resources in these facilities has been associated with the relative distribution (i.e, case mix) of the types of patients under their care, and the beds and services in these facilities are essentially rationed based upon assessments of how efficiently patients can perform basic activities of daily living (such as bathing, dressing, feeding). Increased survival and possible changes in the disease profile of the elderly population leave open the prospect for radical changes in the health and vitality of cohorts reaching older ages in future decades. For instance, on the pessimistic side, it is possible that increased longevity during this era could 1) prolong the period of life during which ADLs are performed less efficiently, possibly as a result of increased exposure to nonlethal debilitating conditions such as arthritis and blindness, 2) alter the disease profile of the population in favor of causes with higher predeath frailty, 3) alter the case mix of elderly patients in acute and long term care facilities in favor of more costly and more debilitating conditions, and 4) increase the demands for and costs of long-term and acute care facilities beyond that expected from present age-specific utilization rates. On the optimistic side, it is possible that we may experience 1) a postponement of the age of first permanent infirmity and a compression of the time period available for less efficient performance on ADLs into a shorter part of the life span, 2) a slowing of the rate of chronic disease progression and a compression of mortality into a shorter age range closer to the biological limit to life, 3) a change in the case mix of elderly patients in favor of less frail, less debilitating and less costly conditions, and 4) a slowdown in the rate of increase in the demands for and costs of long-term acute care facilities as age-specific morbidity rates decline in the face of projected increases in the numbers of elderly.

The point to be made here is not that either of these extremes in their entirety are inevitable outcomes of the fourth stage of the epidemiologic transition, but that there are some fundamental qualitative features of this stage that make these extremes possible. These qualitative features include, among others, the existence of an upper limit to life imposing possibly very different constraints on longevity, and the potential for a change in the disease profile of the population. To quote Soldo and Manton (1985, p. 314), "the near inevitability of chronic morbidity and disability at advanced ages means that there will be a natural evolution of the mix of services required by an aging population [and] the maturing service needs of an aged population must be taken into account to ensure the long-run fiscal viability of integrated health service systems."

Conclusion

According to the theory of the epidemiologic transition, there are three stages that have been characterized generally by a substitution of degenerative diseases for infectious diseases, and life expectancy at birth reaching approximately 70 years of age in the third stage. Based upon the analysis of mortality, life expectancy, and survival data for the United States from the turn of the century to 1980, and projections to the year 2020, the United States appears to have recently entered a fourth stage in the epidemiologic transition—a stage characterized distinctly by rapid mortality declines in advanced ages that are caused by a postponement of the ages at which degenerative diseases tend to kill. This redistribution of degenerative diseases has been referred to as the "Age of Delayed Degenerative Diseases"—a stage that will propel life expectancy into and perhaps beyond eight decades.

These conclusions are based upon mortality projections recently made by the United States Office of the Actuary—projections based upon an extrapolation of cause-specific mortality rates that were observed in recent years. The use of alternative mortality projection models has demonstrated that even small changes in assumptions can produce relatively large differences in projections of life expectancy (Olshansky 1985). It is therefore suggested that the data presented here should be considered cautiously with regard to projections of the pace and extent of prospective mortality declines in advanced ages. Since other research that has been based upon alternative mortality projection models and assumptions indicate that mortality declines may be greater than those projected by the United States Office of the Actuary (Olshansky 1985), it is possible that the pace of mortality declines may not taper off as quickly as the data presented here indicate. At present, we are unable to determine just how long this era of delayed degenerative diseases will last.

The inevitability of the growth of the elderly population, whether it is caused by larger cohorts moving into advanced ages and/or greater proportions of these cohorts surviving to advanced ages as mortality continues to decline, is certain to have a profound influence on the health care industry and social service programs for the elderly in the coming decades. Whether the influence will be positive or negative has yet to be determined. It is suggested in this paper that the age of delayed degenerative diseases represents an unexpected and perhaps welcome era in our epidemiologic history, an era that requires new ways of thinking about aging, disease, morbidity, mortality, and certainly how life will be lived in advanced ages in the very near future.

Bibliography

Arriaga, E. 1984. "Measuring and Explaining the Change in Life Expectancy." *Demography* 21(1):83–96.

Cameron, J. M. 1985. "Case-mix and Resource Use in Long-term Care." *Medical Care* 23(4):296–311.

Chen, M. M., D. P. Wagner. 1978. "Gains in Mortality From Biomedical Research 1930–1975: An Initial Assessment." *Social Science and Medicine* 49(4):509–538.

Crimmins, E. 1984. "Life Expectancy and the Older Population." *Research on Aging* 6(4):490–514.

Cutler, R. G. 1975. "Evolution of Human Longevity and the Genetic Complexity Governing the Aging Rate." *Proceedings of the National Academy of Sciences* 77(11):4664–4668.

Dublin, L. I., A. J. Lotka, M. Spiegelman. 1949. "The Life Table as a Record of Progress to the End of the 19th Century." In *Length of Life*, 26–43. Ronald Press Co., New York.

Faber, J. F. 1982. "Life Tables for the United States: 1900– 2050." Social Security Administration. Actuaries Study No. 87, SSA Pub. No. 11-11534.

Feldman, J. 1983. "Work Ability of the Aged Under Conditions of Improving Mortality." *Milbank Memorial Fund Quarterly/Health and Society* 61(3):430–44.

Fries, J. F. 1980. "Aging, Natural Death, and the Compression of Morbidity." *New England Journal of Medicine* 303:130–35.

Fries, J. F. 1984. "The Compression of Morbidity: Miscellaneous Comments About a Theme." *The Gerontologist* 24(4):354–59.

Fries, J. F., R. Crapo. 1981. *Vitality and Aging.* San Francisco, Calif.: W. H. Freeman & Co.

Gillum, R. F., A. R. Folsom, H. Blackburn. 1984. "Decline in Coronary Heart Disease Mortality: Old Questions and New Facts." *The American Journal of Medicine* 76:1055–1065.

Gruenberg, E. M. 1977. "The Failure of Success." *Milbank Memorial Fund Quarterly* 55:3–24.

Havighurst, R., G. A. Sacher. 1977. "Prospects for Lengthening Life and Vigor." In *Extending the Human Life Span: Social Policy and Social Ethics*, B. Neugarten and R. Havighurst, eds., pp. 13–18. University of Chicago Press.

Havlick, R. J., M. Feinleib, eds. 1979. Proceedings of the Conference on the Decline in Coronary Heart Disease Mortality. U.S. Department of Health, Education and Welfare. Public Health Service. NIH Pub. No. 79–1610.

Hayflick, L. 1982. "Biological Aspects of Aging." In *Biological and Social Aspects of Mortality and the Length of Life*, S. H. Preston, ed. International Union for Scientific Study of Population (IUSSP). Liege, Belgium: Ordina Editions, pp. 223–58.

Kramer, M. 1980. "The Rising Pandemics of Mental Disorders and Associated Chronic Diseases and Disabilities." In *Epidemiologic Research as a Basis for the Organization of Extramural Psychiatry*. Acta Psychiatrica Scandinavica (Supplementum) 285(62):382–97.

Lopez, A. D., K. Hanada. 1982. "Mortality Patterns and Trends Among the Elderly in Developed Countries." *World Health Statistics Quarterly* 35(314):203–24.

Manton, J. G. 1982. "Changing Concepts of Morbidity and Mortality in the Elderly Population." *Milbank Memorial Fund Quarterly/Health and Society* 60(2):183–244.

———. 1984. "Mortality Patterns in Developed Countries." *Comparative Social Research* 7:259–86.

Manton, K. G., B. J. Soldo. 1985. "Dynamics of Health Changes in the Oldest Old: New Perspectives and Evidence." *Milbank Memorial Fund Quarterly/Health and Society* 63(2):206–85.

McCall, N. 1984. "Utilization and Costs of Medicare Services by Beneficiaries in Their Last Year of Life." *Medical Care* 22(4):329–43.

McKinlay, J. B., S. M. McKinlay. 1977. "The Questionable Contribution of Medical Measures to the Decline of Mortality in the United States in the Twentieth Century." *Milbank Memorial Fund Quarterly/Health and Society* 55(3):405–28.

McKinlay, J. B., S. M. McKinlay, S. Jennings, K. Grant. 1983. "Mortality, Morbidity, and the Inverse Care Law." In *Cities and Sickness*, A. L. Greer and S. Greer, eds. Beverly Hills, Calif.: Sage Publications.

Minaker, K. L., J. Rowe. 1985. "Health and Disease Among the Oldest Old: A Clinical Perspective." *Milbank Memorial Fund Quarterly/Health and Society* 63(2):324–49.

Myers, G. C. 1982. "The Aging of Populations." In *International Perspectives on Aging: Population and Policy Challenges*. UNFPA, Policy Development Studies, No. 7. pp. 1–40.

Myers, G. C. 1983. "Mortality Declines, Life Extension and Population Aging." International Population Conference, Manila 1981. IUSSP, Vol. 5, pp. 691–703.

Myers, G. C., K. G. Manton. 1984. "Compression of Mortality: Myth or Reality?" *The Gerontologist* 24(4):346–53.

National Center for Health Statistics. 1963. "Vital Statistics of the United States: 1960." U.S. Department of Health, Education and Welfare. Vol. II–Mortality, Part A.

———. 1974, "Vital Statistics of the United States: 1970." U.S. Department of Health, Education and Welfare. Vol. II–Mortality, Part A (HRA) 75–1101.

———. 1985. "Vital Statistics of the United States: 1980." U.S. Department of Health and Human Services. Vol. II–Mortality, Part A, DHHS Pub. No. (PHS) 85–1101.

Olshansky, S. J. 1984. "The Demographic Effects of Declining Mortality in the United States: A Prospective Analysis." Paper presented at the meetings of the Population Association of America, Minneapolis, Minnesota.

———. 1985. "Pursuing Longevity: Delay vs. Elimination of Degenerative Diseases." *American Journal of Public Health* 75(7):754–57.

Omran, A. R. 1971. "The Epidemiologic Transition: A Theory of the Epidemiology of Population Change." *Milbank Memorial Fund Quarterly* 49(4):509–38.

Palmore, E. 1986. "Trends in the Health of the Aged." *The Gerontologist*. In press.

Pisa, Z., K. Uemura. 1982. "Trends of Mortality From Ischemic Heart Disease and Other Cardiovascular Diseases in 27 Countries, 1968–1977." *World Health Statistics Quarterly* 35(1): 11-47.

Rice, D. P., J. J. Feldman. 1983. "Living Longer in the United States: Demographic Changes and Health Needs of the Elderly." *Milbank Memorial Fund Quarterly/Health and Society* 61(3):362–96.

Rosenwaike, I., N. Yaffe, P. C. Sagi. 1980. "The Recent Decline in Mortality of the Extreme Aged: An Analysis of Statistical Data." *American Journal of Public Health* 70(10):1074–1080.

Schneider, E., J. Brody. 1983. "Aging, Natural Death, and the Compression of Morbidity: Another View." *New England Journal of Medicine* 11:854–55.

Siegel, J. 1979. "Prospective Trends in the Size and Structure of the Elderly Population, Impact of Mortality Trends, and Some Implications." Current Population Reports. U.S. Bureau of the Census. Series P-23, no. 78, pp. 16–18.

Siegel, J. S. 1980. "On the Demography of Aging." *Demography* 17:345-364.

Siegel, J. S., S. L. Hoover. 1984. "International Trends and Perspectives: Aging." U.S. Bureau of the Census, International Research Document No. 12, ISP–RD–12.

Soldo, B. J., K. G. Manton. 1985. "Changes in the Health Status and Service Needs of the Oldest Old: Current Patterns and Future Trends." Milbank Memorial Fund Quarterly/Health and Society 63(2):286–323.

Uemura, K., Z. Pisa. 1985. "Recent Trends in Cardiovascular Disease Mortality in 27 Industrialized Countries." *World Health Statistics Quarterly* 38(2):142–62.

U.S. Bureau of the Census. 1975. *Historical Statistics of the United States. Colonial Times to 1970.* U.S. Department of Commerce, Part I.

U.S. Department of Health, Education and Welfare. 1982. *Health Status Trends.* Public Health Service. DHHS (PHS) pub. no. 82–50157.

U.S. Department of Health and Human Services. 1980. *Cancer Patient Survival Experience.* Public Health Service. NIH pub. no. 80–2148.

U.S. Department of Health and Human Services. 1981. *Report of the Working Group on Arteriosclerosis.* Washington, D.C. NIH pub. no. 81–2034.

———. 1984. *Changes in Mortality Among the Elderly: United States, 1940–1978.* DHHS pub. no. (PHS) 84–1406a.

Verbrugge, L. 1984. "Longer Life but Worsening Health? Trends in Health and Mortality of Middle-Aged and Older Persons." *Milbank Memorial Fund Quarterly/ Health and Society* 62(3):475–519.

Walker, W. J. 1977. "Changing United States Life-style and Declining Vascular Mortality: Cause or Coincidence?" *New England Journal of Medicine* 297:163–65.

Watkins, L. O. 1984. "Why are Death Rates from Coronary Heart Disease Decreasing? Which Preventive Measures are Effective?" *Postgraduate Medicine* 75(8):201–14.

Wiley, J. A., T. C. Camacho. 1980. "Life-style and Future Health Evidence from the Alameda County Study." *Preventive Medicine* 9:1–21.

Comments

Suzanne Dandoy

DR. OLSHANSKY has summarized for us, in an excellent way, data indicating that life expectancies in the United States will increase primarily due to extending the lives of persons already in the older age groups. He talks about what is commonly referred to as "the aging of the aged." Since I am not a statistician or demographer, I will not comment on Dr. Olshansky's use of actuarial data.

However, I would like to differ with his use of epidemiologic terms. He states that prevalence is a product of the incidence rate and the size and age distribution of the population. Actually, prevalence is a product of incidence times the average duration that a disease lasts in an individual. Prevalence is the rate and, therefore, is independent of the size of the population. This rate may be expressed for a specific segment of the population, such as a specific age group. Dr. Olshansky uses the word "morbidity" to mean "illness." However, to most epidemiologists, "morbidity rates" mean "incidence rates." He states that decreases in death rates may be accompanied by decreases in the severity or rate of progression of chronic diseases, thus leading to a reduction in the incidence rate of morbidity (illness). Incidence rates measure the initial occurrence of a disease and have nothing to do with its severity or progression. This use of terms leads Dr. Olshansky to the conclusion that decreases in mortality rates among cohorts actually have some effect on the incidence of disease. In reality, these are independent phenomena.

I would like to identify the degenerative and man-made diseases referenced in Dr. Olshansky's paper as important in the third and fourth stages of the epidemiologic transition. In persons over age 65 years, the chief killers, in order of incidence, are ischemic heart disease (the lack of blood supply to the heart as evidenced by heart attacks), and other forms of heart disease; malignant neoplasms, particularly of the digestive system and the genital system; strokes, especially in the age group 75 and older; pneumonia and influenza; chronic obstructive pulmonary disease; kidney disease; and accidents. Obviously, many of these conditions result from deterioration of the major systems of the body. Many are influenced by the habits and patterns of our lifestyle and so may be called "the man-made diseases."

While these are the major killers of elderly people and, therefore, the conditions for which we are extending the actual age of death, the diseases that impair daily functioning are somewhat different. Forty-five percent of men age 65 or older report that they are limited in a major activity of living due to health problems. Thirty-five percent of women report such limitations. These percentages come from the National Health Interview Survey and did not change in the 22-year period from 1958 to 1980. The leading health problems in both sexes are arthritis, hearing impairments, hypertension, heart disease, chronic sinusitis, varicose veins, and vision impairments. Only two of these problems, heart disease and hypertension, are related to the leading causes of death mentioned earlier. What we have is another set of health problems, in addition to those that cause death, to be addressed in elderly persons. Health problems that account for sickness and limitations on activity are seldom represented singly. Rather, most older persons have a multiplicity of health problems.

Returning to Dr. Olshansky's paper, in Table 2.3 we have seen that the largest gains in temporary life expectancy occurred in the 20-year period from 1930 to 1950—the time when we were finally controlling the infectious diseases through immunization and the use of antibiotics. Improvements in temporary life expectancy accelerated again in the 1970s. I would postulate that these improvements resulted from the increased accessibility to medical care made possible by the Medicare and Medicaid programs, both of which were inaugurated in 1965.

Declining mortality in this country is really influenced by three factors: first, practices that prevent the development of disease; second, improved methods of treating disease; and third, increased availability and use of the health care system by the people. In relation to the topic of this two-day conference, I would suggest that rationing of health care to the elderly could encompass decreases in any or all of these three factors. In turn, that rationing may reverse the life expectancy trends predicted by Dr. Olshansky.

Preventive services have never been widely used by the elderly. In our society, there is a belief that prevention is something to be practiced only by the young—that by the time one has lived 60 or 70 years, future mortality and morbidity have already been determined. And yet we are also beginning to recognize that, while medical technology may delay death, it does not necessarily improve life. Preventive activities, such as regular exercise, improved nutrition, maintaining dentition, and useful pastimes, improve the days as well as lengthen the years that people live. Yet budget allocations require us to concentrate our efforts on preventive activities for the young because, as we say, we can affect a greater number of healthy years of life. In so doing, we condemn the elderly to live without the knowledge and practices that could make them more comfortable and better able to function. Rationing of preventive services is seldom recognized, but does exist.

We can also ration the development of techniques to diagnose and treat disease. The major emphasis of research and advancement in the health care system in the past 25 years has been on early detection and subsequent treatment, what the epidemiologists call "secondary prevention." We can decide that, through this type of rationing, we want to curtail the projected life expectancies predicted by Dr. Olshansky. He has stated that over half of all females born in the year 2020 are expected to survive to their 85th birthday. Much of that remarkable life expectancy will be due to our ability to replace hearts, remove breasts, treat diabetics, and diagnose brain tumors with CAT scans. But how many of these 85-year-old women will have debilitating arthritis or Alzheimer's disease? I heard a group of middle-aged women groan and protest when told that they might very well live into their 80s. Are we doing them a favor or a disservice by developing medical techniques that prolong lives, when we know so little about how to improve the quality of those lives? Should our emphasis in health care research be directed away from the life-saving technologies that only delay mortality, and into life-improving techniques?

Finally, rationing can be directed at the availability and accessibility of health care services. I mentioned earlier that increases in life expectancies in the 1970s might have been due to the Medicaid and Medicare programs that made medical care more accessible. In this third type of rationing, we might continue the development of all types of technology, but limit their use only to persons below age 50, or some other age. Certainly, there is a history of this type of rationing in our country and elsewhere, and this approach will be discussed at length by the other speakers in this conference. Dr. Olshansky's predictions are based on the assumption that this type of rationing will not occur. He predicts that degenerative diseases will remain the major causes of death, but that we will continue to delay these deaths into older ages. This delay in deaths will occur only if we continue to make all health care services available to the elderly.

In a 1983 survey by the Policy Research Institute and Project HOPE, 415 health system leaders in the United States were asked questions concerning their expectations for trends in health status in the next 20 years. They felt that life expectancy would continue to increase. These leaders credited medical technology as most responsible for past gains, but thought that lifestyle changes would most influence future changes in life expectancy. Interestingly, they also thought that lifestyle was the chief factor contributing to the deterioration in health status in the last 20 years. Apparently, they thought that people in the United States had awakened to the need to take more responsibility for their health status and would, in fact, change their lifestyles.

In discussing the implications of his findings, Dr. Olshansky mentions two options: that declining mortality in advanced ages may result in additional years of health, or that it may produce additional years of frailty and senescence. He concludes that morbidity will also be postponed into more advanced ages so that the elderly will have more years of health. I cannot agree. We do not have evidence indicating that significant improvements have been or will be made in those conditions causing elderly people to be severely limited in their physical and mental activities. In fact, improved survival of persons already with chronic diseases and impairments will give them more time to develop other illnesses and for their present illnesses to become more severe.

Until we can ease more of the pain from arthritis, prevent or correct more hearing and vision problems, and delay the onset of mental deterioration and confusion, we may force increasing numbers of elderly citizens to spend more years dependent on their aging children or confined to institutional facilities.

The changes outlined in Dr. Olshansky's presentation have profound effects on the health care delivery system, the age at which we cause people to retire, the way in which we approach additional advances in medical technology, and how we prepare ourselves and our children to handle an increasingly older population. The challenges are apparent and should serve to stimulate considerable discussion.

3

Memory Processes in the Aged

Gary Gillund

Introduction

O<small>LSHANSKY HAS PRESENTED EVIDENCE</small> that indicates a trend toward increased longevity among older cohorts and has suggested that this trend will continue to influence our population in the immediate future. In this chapter, I will describe the cognitive functioning of older adults and project what changes in cognitive functioning may result from an increase in the length of old age.

Cognitive functions include processes such as attention, perception, memory, problem solving, decision-making, and intelligence. To review all these processes is well beyond the scope of this paper. Instead, I will selectively review the literature on memory functioning.

The choice of memory functioning can be justified at several levels. First, it is obvious that memory problems are of primary concern to many older adults. Memory problems are commonly reported by the elderly, and most of us believe that our memories will worsen with increasing age (Hulick 1982; Perlmutter 1978). Second, memory is an important component of several other cognitive functions. In many accounts of intelligence (Horn 1982), problem solving (Arenberg 1982; Rabbitt 1977), language comprehension (Burke and Light 1981), and reading (Kintsch and van Dijk 1978), memory plays a significant role in determining overall performance. Therefore, an understanding of

This work was supported by BRSG Grant No. S07 RR07092 awarded by the Biomedical Research Support Grant Program, Division of Health Resources, National Institutes of Health, to the University of Utah. Direct correspondence to Gary Gillund, Department of Psychology, University of Utah, Salt Lake City, Utah 84112.

memory processes may facilitate an understanding of more complex processes. Finally, among older adults, memory is composed of a complex set of processes that are related to several important applications. For example, memory loss is one of the earliest symptoms of Alzheimer's disease (Petit 1982), and other changes in health are often related to memory problems (Siegler and Costa 1985). Because of the plasticity (modifiability) of certain memory processes, there is a growing concern with improving the memory capabilities of older adults with training programs (Baltes and Willis 1982).

The remainder of this chapter is devoted to a brief review of the literature on memory and aging, a discussion of some of the causes of memory decline in old age, and some predictions for the influence of an increase in the length of old age on memory function.

Unless specifically noted, I will refer to adults between the ages of 60 and 80 years of age as "older adults" for the remainder of this chapter.

Memory Across Adulthood

Memory is a system of structures and processes that are influenced by characteristics of the individual, the to-be-remembered material, the conditions of learning, and the conditions at test (Jenkins 1979). These factors do not combine in a simple fashion to determine memory performance, but rather interact in a complex manner. The complexity in determining memory performance makes general statements about the effects of age on memory difficult at best. However, there appear to be at least three critical findings that all serious approaches to memory and aging must address. First, most studies of memory, and cognitive processes in general, show a significant decline in performance associated with age. Second, the rate of decline varies widely from task to task; some tasks show large declines associated with age, while a few tasks actually reveal superior performance by older adults. Third, the decline associated with age also varies widely with individuals. Some individuals begin to show a decline relatively early in life, whereas others reveal virtually no decline until very late in life, if at all. This chapter will try to address these three issues within three general areas of research interest: processing resources, knowledge structures, and individual differences.

Processing Resources

"Processing resources" are the mechanisms of memory functioning. They are the means with which we deal with information. These resources are critical components of all stages of memory functioning.

Some examples of processing resources include the speed with which we can deal with information, the ability or amount of attention we can allocate to relevant information, and the amount of information (capacity) we can deal with at any given time. These and related processing resources have been found to decline in efficiency with increasing age, although the onset and rate of decline have been found to vary widely. (See Craik and Byrd 1982 for a discussion of attention; see Salthouse 1985 for a discussion of speed of processing; and see Talland 1968 for a discussion of capacity.) The relative role of each of these factors is not well specified, however. In fact, few theories exist that describe the role of a single factor on aging in any detail, much less describe the relationship between these factors. Therefore, I will simply describe these theoretically separable processes as if they all contribute to a general factor that I will label "processing resources."

There are three reasons why a discussion of processing resources is important for a discussion of cognitive processes and aging. First, virtually all cognitive tasks make use of processing resources, and there is a great deal of evidence that processing resources decline in efficiency with age (Craik and Byrd 1982; Salthouse 1985). Therefore, the decline in efficiency of processing resources may go a long way in explaining the deficits exhibited by the elderly on most memory tasks. Second, another important factor to consider is that not all memory tests are equally demanding of processing resources. Some tasks require a great deal of processing resources (e.g., trying to remember the names of twenty new acquaintances at a party), while others require very little effort and thus demand little of processing resources (e.g., trying to remember your name). Thus, as we increase task difficulty by increasing the demand on processing resources, we expect that age differences will increase, and there is a good deal of evidence that supports this contention (Birren, Rigel, and Morrison 1982; Brinley 1965; Canestrari 1963). Third, the loss of processing resources is not inconsistent with physiological changes that occur with age. While the exact relationship between physiological processes and psychological processes is far from well specified, the idea of a loss of mental energy or speed is quite consistent with physical changes that occur in other bodily functions. (See Poon 1985 for a discussion.) Therefore, if one assumes that there are individual differences in the aging process, and there are certainly individual changes in the occurrence of disease, then to the degree that these changes parallel changes in processing resources, some of the variability in performance on cognitive tasks may be explained.

To summarize, an understanding of processing resources is important for an understanding of age changes in cognition, because a decline in processing resources may, in large part, be responsible for the commonly reported decline on many cognitive tasks with age. In addition, because different tasks place different demands on processing resources, age differences will vary with task demands. Finally, to the degree that the loss of processing resources are reflected in physiological changes with age and disease, we may begin to explain some of the variability found between subjects. However, a loss in efficiency of processing resources explains neither why some tasks are more demanding of processing resources than others, nor does it explain all the variability found between subjects. To address these issues, we need to discuss knowledge structures.

Knowledge Structures

The second factor that I believe is critical for explaining the effects of age on memory is knowledge structures. Knowledge structures include both the amount of information one has in a particular domain and the way that the information is organized (Chi 1978). Knowledge structures can vary in complexity from simple associations between pairs of words (Raaijmakers and Shiffrin 1981) to detailed outlines or summaries of complex activities like attending a restaurant (Bower, Black and Turner 1979). Knowledge structures aid both encoding and retrieval processes.

When information is encoded, the processes do not occur in a vacuum. We use our knowledge structures to give meaning to incoming material. In general, the more knowledge we have about a given topic, the easier it is to encode new information relevant to that knowledge (Chase and Simon 1973; Chi 1978). For example, it is much easier for an individual who has stored in memory the rules, regulations, and general structure of a baseball game to remember the events that transpire during a game than an individual who does not have such knowledge (Chiesi, Spilich and Voss 1979).

Knowledge structures may guide our attention, provide us with ways to organize or group incoming information, and lead us to expect certain events. Additionally, because structures result in relatively easy encoding of information that is directly related to existing knowledge structures, they may free up processing resources so that more time or attention can be given to unexpected or novel information (Anderson and Pichert 1978).

Knowledge structures also facilitate retrieval processes. Knowledge structures may serve as cues to locate relevant material in memory. For example, if asked to recall the events that transpired during a particular baseball game, knowledge that nine innings are played and that three outs per team are awarded each inning serves as a starting point to search for specific types of events that occurred during the game. A knowledge structure may serve to generate plausible instances that will be checked for their occurrence during the particular event being recalled (Rabinowitz, Mandler and Barsalou 1979).

Knowledge structures do not appear to deteriorate with age. Whether the structures are simple, such as word meanings (Horn and Cattell 1966) and word associations (Howard, McAndrews and Lasaga 1981), or very complex like schemata for everyday activities (Light and Anderson 1983), the structures of adults do not disappear or become less functional with age. However, it is possible, or even likely, that the types of structures employed in everyday activities may be different for younger and older adults, because structures tend to develop that are useful in dealing with everyday environmental situations (Perlmutter, 1986). Therefore, when comparing younger and older adults' memory performance, it is important to control or manipulate the relevance of the to-be-remembered materials to the knowledge structures of both age groups. If materials or tasks are chosen so that they are more meaningful to younger adults in terms of the knowledge structures they access, then age differences will appear that are not due to the aging process per se, but rather to a materials bias.

I have argued that knowledge structures may facilitate encoding and retrieval and that knowledge structures do not appear to decline in effectiveness with increasing age. In addition, knowledge structures may partially compensate for a loss of processing resources in several ways. Knowledge structures may allow individuals to eliminate certain stages of processing. For example, suppose a subject is asked if a touchdown occurred during a particular baseball game. If the subject has no knowledge of sports, then a search of all the terms and events announced during the game has to be checked to determine if a touchdown appeared at any time. On the other hand, a knowledge of sports would allow the subject to skip the searches and reject the touchdown on the basis that a touchdown is a football activity and thus could not have occurred during a baseball game.

Knowledge structures can also reduce the amount of information that has to be dealt with at any given time. That is, structures can be used to group information and effectively reduce the amount of information that needs to be processed, thus reducing processing demand. For example, a knowledge of historical events allows "17761812192919731985" to be coded as "1776, 1812, 1929, 1973, 1985," thus reducing the material to be remembered from twenty numbers to five and, in addition, making the numbers more meaningful.

Finally, there is evidence that some very well learned semantic structures may come to be processed automatically (without awareness), and thus demand a minimum of processing resources (Schneider and Shiffrin 1977).

In all these cases, the constraints put on older adults by a decrease in processing resources can be at least partially compensated for by a well-developed knowledge structure. However, it is probably the case that even a well-developed knowledge structure does not compensate for extreme processing demands. For example, Charness (1981) selected older and younger adults who were comparable in chess ability (and presumably chess-knowledge structures); they were asked to recall chess positions of actual games after being presented for only five seconds. Age differences favored younger adults. Thus, in this case, the knowledge structure was not sufficient to compensate for the effects of loss of processing resources.

To summarize, knowledge structures greatly facilitate the processing of information. There is little evidence to suggest that the structures disappear or somehow decline in efficiency with age, and therefore knowledge structures do not facilitate an understanding of the typically reported age decline in cognitive performance. However, if tasks are chosen such that the materials are relevant to young adults' knowledge structures but not to older adults' structures, then differences between the groups might mistakenly be attributed to age when, in fact, age is not the critical variable. In addition, knowledge structures may compensate for a loss of processing resources. Compared to tasks where subjects have little familiarity (few knowledge structures), age differences on tasks where subjects have a good deal of familiarity will be much reduced.

Finally, this account is not a new one in many respects. The idea that both structures and processes must be specified in any account of memory performance has been known for some time (Anderson 1976). Also, in the area of intelligence and aging, research has shown that verbal and general information types of knowledge (experience dependent knowledge) do not decline with age, but other processes that are not dependent on experience do show declines. (See Horn's 1982 discussion of fluid and crystallized intelligence for an example.)

Individual Differences

One of the biggest problems in describing age changes in memory processes is the incredible interindividual variability in memory performance. Among college students, individual differences in verbal ability, for example, appear to be responsible for qualitative as well as quantitative differences in memory performance (Hunt 1985). In addition, individual differences appear to increase with increasing age (Thomae 1979). Almost all memory studies find a larger variance score for older adults than for younger adults. This increase in variation is probably due to wider variations in current health status, cumulative effects of differing health problems, educational experiences, socioeconomic histories, and different rates of aging that are genetically determined.

In most studies of memory, college students are compared to adults between the ages of 60 and 80. Distributions of memory performance scores for these two age groups reveal two important differences. First, if the mean performance of the two groups of subjects is compared, age differences favoring young adults are found. In fact, most studies of memory have found age differences favoring young adults. On the other hand, for any given level of performance, one can find older adults who will perform equivalently to younger adults. For example, many researchers have found that when younger and older individuals are matched on verbal ability (i.e., both groups can be classified as high verbal), age differences in memory performance disappear (Barrett and Wright 1981; Bowles and Poon 1982; Cavanaugh 1983; Craik and Masani 1967; Gillund and Perlmutter 1985; Hess 1984; Till 1985). Other individual difference variables that have been found to reduce or eliminate age differences in memory performance include health, education, and intelligence. In general, in most studies in which a sufficiently large number of subjects are tested, some older adults are found to perform as well as the best performing younger adults.

To summarize, when the performance on a memory task of a sample of older adults is compared to a sample of younger adults, age differences typically are found favoring the younger adults. However, there are large individual differences found within all age groups, and these differences appear to increase with age. Even at advanced ages, some proportion of older adults perform as well as the best younger adults.

Individual differences add to the difficulty of describing general changes in memory performance with age. Age declines may be virtually nonexistent for some older adults. On the other hand, most older adults show a decline in the efficiency of cognitive processes, although the loss is selective. At the other extreme, some older adults who are in poor health often reveal a debilitating loss of cognitive function across virtually all domains of cognitive performance. Fortunately, this latter group is still in the minority.

Aging and Memory: Present and Future

In this section, I will provide a description of memory performance across adulthood and discuss how this description might change as more adults reach old age and live more of their lives as old adults.

Before an attempt is made to provide such a description, some cautionary notes are provided. The description below is speculative. Hard data on age changes in very late life are rare. Furthermore, projections based on current data are difficult at best. Therefore, I will simply outline some factors that are likely to be of importance in determining what changes in cognitive processes of older adults might be observed in the future.

The Old-Old

The research I have summarized has been primarily directed at adults between the ages of 60 and 80. A question arises as to whether the generalizations presented in this paper are applicable to those adults over age 80 (the old-old). This question is extremely important because this age group is the fastest growing segment of our population. Unfortunately, there is little data on adults over the age of 80. However, existing data suggest that results do not generalize very well to the old-old. At some point in the life span (on the average 80 years of age, although the variability is quite large), we see a sharp decline in a number of cognitive functions. That is, processing resources show a sharp drop in efficiency, much sharper than the slow decline that is revealed across earlier adulthood. In addition, it appears that the ability to compensate for the decline with the employment of knowledge structures is also greatly diminished very late in life. Whether this results from an actual decline of the efficiency of the structures, or whether the loss of processing resources is so great that structures simply are not as useful is not clear, but the practical result is that performance declines sharply.

The increase in the proportion of the old-old in our population would appear to contribute to a higher incidence of declining cognitive functioning among the elderly. However, the exact form of this impact will depend on a number of factors including general health, the presence of certain diseases, and the effectiveness of training programs.

General Health

The exact changes that occur in memory processing in a large proportion of the population achieving old age depends in large part on the relative frequency of individual difference variables. For example, changes in health status are likely to have a significant impact on normative changes in memory performance. The presence of chronic diseases increases with age. Some researchers estimate that as many as 86 percent of all adults over the age of 65 have at least one chronic health problem (Satariano and Syme 1981). In addition, approximately 20 percent of these people have two or more chronic diseases, and 33 percent have three or more. Of course, not all of these diseases influence memory performance directly. However, some health problems, like hypertension, are highly correlated with memory performance and show an increase in incidence with increasing age. In addition, health problems may have a cumulative effect on memory performance. Small amounts of damage may build up and not manifest themselves until some critical amount of damage has been done. With increasing age, adults are more likely to reach that critical stage.

Based on this line of reasoning, memory problems should become more frequent as the age of the population increases. However, this argument ignores changes that might result from advances in medicine, diet, lifestyle, and education. For example, between 1950 and 1978, the rate of death due to heart disease dropped by 20 percent, and the rate of death due to stroke dropped by almost 60 percent (Levy and Moskowitz 1982). As medical treatment improves, and an awareness that exercise, diet, and lifestyle may increase the probability of avoiding those health problems, the rates may continue to decline. Thus, there may be a tradeoff between an increase in diseases with increasing age and a decrease in the incidence and impact of disease due to improvements in medical treatment and lifestyles. The exact nature of the tradeoff is, of course, unknown. Also unknown is whether improved health will simply postpone the cognitive decline, or whether it might actually reduce the decline.

Dementia

The presence of Alzheimer's disease and related diseases that primarily influence the elderly is a dark cloud over this analysis. While there are several diseases that have similar effects on the cognitive functioning of the elderly, I will briefly mention Alzheimer's disease because of its prevalence, and because it is being widely studied. At the present time, Alzheimer's disease affects approximately 5 percent of the population over age 65. However, the incidence of the disease increases in individuals up to age 85 and then appears to level off or even decrease slightly (Hagnell, Lanke, Rorsman, and Ojesjo 1981). In addition, if deaths due to heart disease, stroke, and cancer were eliminated, perhaps more of these people might contract Alzheimer's disease in later life. If life expectancy reaches the late 90s, and other diseases become less common, some researchers estimate that as much as 45 percent of the population would develop Alzheimer's disease (Terry and Katzman 1983). These individuals would show relatively rapid and severe declines in memory performance as well as in all other cognitive processes. If, in fact, there is an increase in the incidence of dementia with increasing age, the normative cognitive functioning would be expected to decline in the future.

Education

There is some evidence that cognitive processes maintained throughout adulthood do not show as rapid declines as those processes that are not frequently employed (Perlmutter 1978). While the boundary conditions for this effect are not known, and while it may be that this effect serves primarily to postpone the decline or slow the decline rather than prevent it, it may prove a fruitful area of further research.

Remediation

If we assume that typical older adults will reveal cognitive deficits with increasing age, then an important question is whether we can do anything to alleviate the deficit. One method that is receiving considerable attention is the training of older adults in certain mnemonics or cognitive strategies. In general, these training programs have been found to facilitate older adults' performance in tasks such as word recall (Poon, Walsh-Sweeney and Fozard 1980), face/name learning (Yesavage, Rose and Bower 1983), and some measures of intelligence (Baltes and Willis 1982). While older adults do appear to benefit from the training, a note of caution is warranted. As Poon (1985) has suggested, all people do not benefit from the training, the techniques do not work in all situations, and the maintenance of the benefit over time has yet to be demonstrated.

Another approach that has received much less attention is the use of external memory aids such as notes and diaries. B.F. Skinner (1983) has presented some of these aids in an anecdotal fashion. While such aids may appear trivial, they are quite useful because they greatly reduce memory demands. In addition, effective use of the aids can be learned. For example, if you discover from the evening news that there is a high probability of rain the next day, then a useful strategy is to immediately (so you will not forget to do it) hang your umbrella on the door where it will serve as a cue to remember to carry it with you the following day. The usefulness of such aids is now being recognized by several businesses that supply, for example, pill boxes that contain programmable clocks that beep when a drug should be administered. While this area of research is very new, it would appear to be a promising area for future inquiry.

Conclusions

It should be clear from this paper that general conclusions regarding aging and cognition are extremely difficult. Some older adults reveal virtually no declines in cognitive processes with increasing age. Others, who may have some form of dementia, show a rapid and severe loss of cognitive function. The large majority of older adults reveal a selective decline in memory and related functions. The declines for most of us will be on tasks with which we are unfamiliar and that place a heavy demand on our processing resources. On most everyday tasks older adults function quite well.

As our older adults get older, the picture becomes less clear. As we pass the age of 80, our processing resources appear to decline more rapidly and we appear less able to compensate for the loss. In addition, we become more susceptible to several debilitating diseases that further hamper our cognitive functions. On the other hand, as we become aware of the factors that affect cognitive function and as treatments for the diseases become available, we might be able to at least partially offset these limitations. The extent and exact nature of the treatments and preventions on cognitive function, however, remains to be determined.

To summarize, along with the decrease in mortality among the aged predicted by Olshansky, there is likely to be an increase in morbidity. However, two factors should be noted. First, for a significant proportion of the population, the declines will be small or selective. Second, changes in lifestyle, some forms of remediation, and medical advances, especially in the area of dementia, hold the potential for a curtailing of the morbidity.

References

Anderson, J. R. 1976. *Language, Memory, and Thought*. Hillsdale, N.J.: Lawrence Erlbaum Assoc.

Anderson, R. C., J. W. Pichert. 1978. "Recall of Previously Unrecallable Information Following a Shift in Perspective." *Journal of Verbal Learning and Verbal Behavior* 17:1–12.

Arenberg, D. 1982. "Changes with Age in Problem Solving." In *Aging and Cognitive Processes*, F. I. M. Craik and S. Trehub, eds. New York: Plenum Press.

Baltes, P. B. and S. L. Willis. 1982. "Enhancement (plasticity) of Intellectual Functioning: Penn State's Adult Development and Enrichment Projects." (ADEPT) In *Aging and Cognitive Processes*, F. I. M. Craik and S. Trehub, eds. New York: Plenum Press.

Barrett, T. R. and M. Wright 1981. "Age-related Facilitation in Recall Following Semantic Processing." *Journal of Gerontology* 36:194–99.

Birren, J. E., K. F. Riegel and D. F. Morrison. 1962. "Age Differences in Response Speed as a Function of Controlled Variations of Stimulus Conditions: Evidence of a General Speed Factor." *Gerontologia* 6:1–18.

Bower, G. H., J. B. Black and T. J. Turner. 1979. "Scripts in Memory for Text." *Cognitive Psychology* 11; 177–220.

Bowles, N. L. and L. W. Poon. 1982. "An Analysis of the Effect of Aging on Recognition Memory." *Journal of Gerontology* 37:212–19.

Brinley, J. F. 1965. "Cognitive Sets, Speed, and Accuracy of Performance in the Elderly." In *Behavior, Aging and the Nervous System*, A. T. Welford and J. E. Birren, eds. Springfield, Ill.: Charles C. Thomas.

Burke, D. M. and L. L. Light. 1981. "Memory and Aging: The Role of Retrieval Processes." *Psychological Bulletin* 90:513–46.

Canestrari, R. E., Jr. 1963. "Paced and Self-paced Learning in Young and Elderly Adults." *Journal of Gerontology* 18:165–68.

Cavanaugh, J. C. 1983. "Comprehension and Retention of Television Programs by 20- and 60-Year-Olds." *Journal of Gerontology* 38:190–96.

Charness, N. 1981. "Visual Short-term Memory and Aging in Chess Players." *Journal of Gerontology* 36:615–719.

Chase, W. G. and H. A. Simon. 1973. "The Mind's Eye in Chess." In *Visual Information Processing*, W. G. Chase, ed. New York: Academic Press.

Chi, M. T. H. 1978. "Knowledge Structures and Memory Development." In *Children's Thinking: What Develops?*, R. S. Siegler, ed. Hillsdale, N.J.: Lawrence Erlbalm Associates.

Chiesi, H. L., G. J. Spilich and J. F. Voss. 1979. "Acquisition of Domain-related Information in Relation to High and Low Domain Knowledge." *Journal of Verbal Learning and Verbal Behavior* 18:257–73.

Craik, F. I. M. and M. Byrd. 1982. "Aging and Cognitive Deficits: The Role of Attentional Resources." In *Aging and Cognitive Processes*, F. I. M. Craik and S. Trehub, eds. New York: Plenum Press.

Craik, F. I. M. and P. A. Masani. 1967. "Age Differences in the Temporal Integration of Language." *British Journal of Psychology* 58:201–99.

Gillund, G. and M. Perlmutter. 1985. "Recall from Semantic and Episodic Memory." Presented at the American Psychological Association meetings, Toronto, Canada, August 1984. (ERIC Document Reproduction Service No. ED 251–733).

Hagnell, O., J. Lanke, B. Rorsman and L. Ojesjo. 1981. "Does the Incidence of Age Psychosis Decrease?" *Neuropsychobiology* 7:201–11.

Hess, T. M. 1984. "Effects of Semantically Related and Unrelated Contexts on Recognition Memory of Different-aged Adults." *Journal of Gerontology* 39:444–51.

Horn, J. L. and R. B. Cattell. 1966. "Age Differences in Primary Mental Ability Factors." *Journal of Gerontology* 21:210–20.

Horn, J. L. 1982. "The Theory of Fluid and Crystallized Intelligence in Relation to Concepts of Cognitive Psychology and Aging in Adulthood." In *Aging and Cognitive Processes*, F. I. M. Craik and S. Trehub, eds. New York: Plenum Press.

Howard, D. V., M. P. McAndrews and M. I. Lasaga. 1981. "Semantic Priming of Lexical Decisions in Young and Old Adults." *Journal of Gerontology* 36:707–14.

Hulicka, I. M. 1982. "Memory Functioning in Late Adulthood." In *Aging and Cognitive Processes*, F. I. M. Craik and S. Trehab, eds. New York: Plenum Press.

Hunt, E. 1985. "Verbal Ability." In *Human Abilities: An Information Processing Approach*, R. J. Sternberg, ed. New York: W. H. Freeman.

Jenkins, J. J. 1979. "Four Points to Remember: A Tetrahedral Model of Memory." In *Levels of Processing in Human Memory*, L. S. Cermak and F. I. M. Craik, eds. Hillsdale, N.J.: Lawrence Erlbaum Associates.

Kintsch, W. and T. A. van Dijk. 1978. "Toward a Model of Text Comprehension and Production." *Psychological Review* 85:363–94.

Levy, R. I. and J. Moskowitz. 1982. "Cardiovascular Research: Decades of Progress, a Decade of Promise." *Science* 217:121–29.

Light, L. L. and P. A. Anderson. 1983. "Memory for Scripts in Young and Older Adults." *Memory and Cognition* 11:435–44.

Perlmutter, M. 1978. "What is Memory Aging the Aging of?" *Developmental Psychology* 14:330–45.

Perlmutter, M. 1986. "A Life Span View of Memory." In *Advances in Lifespan Development and Behavior, Vol. 7*, P. B. Baltes, D. Featherman, and R. Learner, eds. Hillsdale, N.J.: Lawrence Erlbaum Associates.

Petit, T. L. 1982. "Neuroanatomical and Clinical Neuropsychological Changes in Senile Dementia." In *Aging and Cognitive Processes*, F. I. M. Craik and S. Trehub, eds. New York: Plenum Press.

Poon, L. W. 1985. "Differences in Human Memory with Aging: Nature, Causes, and Clinical Implications." In *Handbook of the Psychology of Aging (2d ed.)*, J. E. Birren and K. W. Schaie, eds. New York: Van Nostrand Reinhold.

Poon, L. W., L. Walsh-Sweeney and J. L. Fozard. 1980. "Memory Skill Training for the Elderly: Salient Issues on the Use of Imagery Mnemonics." In *New Directions in Memory and Aging*, L. W. Poon, J. L. Fozard, L. S. Cermak, D. Arenberg, and L. W. Thompson, eds. Hillsdale, N.J.: Lawrence Erlbaum Associates.

Raaijmakers, J. G. R. and R.M. Shiffrin. 1981. "Search of Associative Memory." *Psychological Review* 88:93–134.

Rabbitt, P. 1977. "Changes in Problem-Solving Ability in Older Age." In *Handbook of the Psychology of Aging*, J. E. Birren and K. W. Schaie, eds. New York: Van Nostrand Reinhold.

Rabinowitz, J. C., G. Mandler and L. W. Barsalou. "Generation-recognition as an Auxiliary Retrieval Strategy." *Journal of Verbal Learning and Verbal Behavior* 18:57–72.

Salthouse, T. A. 1985. "Speed of Behavior and Its Implications for Cognition." In *Handbook of the Psychology of Aging*, J. E. Birren and K. W. Schaie, eds. New York: Van Nostrand Reinhold.

Satariano, W. A. and S. L. Syme. 1981. "Life Changes and Disease in Elderly Populations: Coping with Change." In *Aging: Biology and Behavior*, J. L. McGaugh and S. B. Kiesler, eds. New York: Academic Press.

Schneider, W. and R. M. Shiffrin. 1977. "Controlled and Automatic Human Information Processing: Part 1. Detection, Search, and Attention." *Psychological Review* 84:1–66.

Siegler, I. C. and P. T. Costa, Jr. 1985. "Health Behavior Relationships." In *Handbook of the Psychology of Aging (2d ed.)*, J. E. Birren and K. W. Schaie, eds. New York: Van Nostrand Reinhold.

Skinner, B. F. 1983. "Intellectual Self-management in Old Age." *American Psychologist* 38:239–44.

Talland, G. A. 1968. "Aging and the Span of Immediate Recall." In *Human Aging and Behavior*, G. A. Talland, ed. New York: Academic Press.

Terry, R. D. and R. Katzman. 1983. "Senile Dementia of the Alzheimer Type." *Annals of Neurology* 14:497–506.

Thomae, H. 1979. "The Concept of Development and Life-Span Developmental Psychology." In *Life-span Development and Behavior, Vol. 2*, P. B. Baltes and O. G. Brim, Jr., eds. New York: Academic Press.

Till, R. E. 1985. "Verbatim and Inferential Memory in Young and Elderly Adults." *Journal of Gerontology* 40:316–23.

Yesavage, J. A., T. L. Rose, G. H. Bower. 1983. "Interactive Imagery and Effective Judgments Improve Face-name Learning in the Elderly." *Journal of Gerontology* 38:197–203.

Comments

John L. Horn

Ｈｏｗ ｄｏ ｗｅ ｆｉｔ what we know about human abilities within the context of questions we should consider when we try to understand health care rationing among the elderly? Does it matter whether or not human abilities decline with age, either statistically—on the average, but not necessarily for all—or inevitably in all individuals? Should the ethics, the politics, and the economics of health care rationing remain the same regardless of the answer to this question?

Consider the ethical issues for just a moment. Look at the extremes, for the issues can be most clearly distinguished in their extreme forms. Suppose there is a low level of intellectual ability in a person—any person, not necessarily an elderly one. What are the ethical obligations of that person, and what are the obligations society has to that person?

Notice first that if ability is low enough, the person is, in effect, excluded from the society in which individuals are expected to make ethical decisions. A person of low ability has few ethical obligations and, concomitantly, few of the rights and privileges associated with citizenship. We cannot be crystal clear in statements about the minimum ability below which one is excluded from ethical citizenship, and we are not clear about how we measure this minimum ability. But we know that at some level, ability is too low to enable one to do ethical reasoning, and when we see that extreme, we act on that knowledge: we exclude the testimony of young children; we make decisions about old people because, we argue, the decisions are

Preparation of this manuscript was supported, in part, by grants from the National Institute of Aging (AG04704) and the National Institute of Child Health and Human Development (HD1752).

necessary for the person's own good; we allow a verdict of "not guilty by reason of incompetence" not only in courts of law, but also in many day-to-day decisions. A particular minimum level of intellectual ability is a requisite for ethical citizenship; there is no doubt about this.

What has been said here about ethical citizenship applies to politics and economics; more than a particular minimum level of ability is required to participate in the work force and in citizen activities. A person of sufficiently low ability is excluded from most jobs, and is virtually eliminated entirely from promotional systems. If that person has capital, these resources are usually managed by others. The person's political interests are interpreted and prosecuted by others, not by the person himself.

How do these exclusions apply to the elderly when there is a decline in intellectual ability? The answer is that the exclusions apply in much the same way, but ambiguity is introduced by inertia. We do not change our beliefs easily: if it has been believed that a person is competent, that belief tends to persist—in that person as well as in others—despite evidence indicating that the person's competence has notably waned. For this reason, exclusion rules are sometimes applied somewhat more gingerly to the elderly than to other persons. But given this condition and the problems of defining how low ability has to drop before exclusions are imposed, the exclusions are applied to the elderly in the same way as they are applied to others. The ethical, political, and economic citizenship of the elderly person is revoked when intellectual ability drops, or is believed to have dropped, to a sufficiently low level.

Extreme cases illustrate what is true when the decline of intellectual ability is not necessarily, or not known to be, extreme. Consider economic citizenship, for example. Do the elderly lose important rights of economic participation partly in consequence of beliefs we have about how abilities decline with age, whether or not we have sound evidence for these beliefs? I think the answer to this question is "yes." The elderly are excluded from important areas of economic activity partly because it is widely believed that they are not intellectually capable. This occurs despite notable exceptions (e.g., in selection of political leaders). It occurs even when it is recognized that what is true for some of the elderly is not true for all of them. Retirement policies and practices, for example, are based on the assumption that ability losses occur in a sufficiently large proportion of the elderly population to warrant mandatory retirement for all of that population. In some cases, this amounts to taking a job from a more capable individual and giving it to a less capable individual.

Exclusion of the elderly from economic activities occurs even when there is belief that their abilities are not as low as is required to exclude other humans from the same activity. This seems to come about because there is a belief that the ability deficits of the elderly cannot be corrected, but comparable deficits in the young are remedial—or at last there is hope for the young.

Elderly individuals of relatively high intellectual ability are excluded from jobs on the basis of conspiracies, policies, and laws that would be regarded as unfair if they were applied to other groups, not to mention other minorities. Beliefs about abilities of elderly people are at the core of justifications for these exclusions.

The beliefs on which exclusion decisions are based are often accepted implicitly, without clear justification. Such beliefs can be regarded as irrefutable, universal "facts." The validity of the beliefs often is not questioned. What might have been found to be true for some of the elderly or for the average of an elderly population is accepted as true for all the elderly. Laws ordaining mandatory retirement at age 70, in some jobs, derive, in part, from an implicit assumption that important abilities are lacking in the elderly.

To recognize the powerful and unexamined nature of these beliefs is not to argue that they are never questioned. The beliefs are the basis of laws, rules, and practices, but there are many who question the beliefs. Such questions have been brought to the forum. For example, there have been lawsuits pertaining to the minimum ability required of commercial airplane pilots. Nevertheless, poorly examined beliefs based on common sense have been prominent parts of the evidence accepted in the proceedings.

There is, then, widespread, readily accepted belief that major human abilities decline with age, and this belief is brought into practices that have important consequences, not only for the elderly, but for all people. Belief about the age-linked decline of human abilities is a serious matter. On the basis of such belief, ethical, political, and economic citizenship is taken away from elderly individuals. Is it sensible, is it fair to do this? What is the nature of the evidence that supports the belief? Is this evidence being interpreted properly—in law, in the rules of businesses and the government, and in the practices that determine how elderly people are treated?

I suggest that much of what is accepted as evidence about the abilities of the elderly is simply unsubstantiated but widespread belief. One form of commonly held belief derives from observations of particular cases. Each of us has noticed that a particular person, over the age of 70 years, has dropped to a low level of ability. On this basis, we hastily generalize that people over 70 years of age have low ability. Because this generalization is shared by many, the belief that the elderly have low ability is widely accepted. The implicit assumption seems to be that since many of us have observed the outcome of our particular samples, that outcome of our samples is true for an entire population these samples are assumed to represent. But our samples are not representative of the population to which we generalize, collating the results of such samples (popular meta-analysis, we might call it) cannot make the ultimate result representative. Moreover, even if the meta-analysis did lead to a proper estimation of the population average, it would not be correct to assume that an average represents all individuals of the class on which that average is based.

Hasty generalization from unrepresentative samples and over-generalization from an assumed average are ubiquitous errors of human reasoning. Laws, rules, and practices that restrict the elderly are based on such errors. These errors appear in the rationale for laws about retirement, for example. Retirement laws (the 1978 Age Discrimination and Employment Act) stipulate that in particular occupations (judges excuse themselves from application of the law), each and every person must retire at age 70. In justifying the law, it is argued that the elderly do not perform as well on the job as do the youthful. But the evidence put forth to support this statement is based on the average for the elderly and the average for the youthful: an average does not represent the many people scoring above (among the elderly) and below (among the youthful) the average. Powerful policy decisions about the elderly have been based on this kind of defective evidence.

It is true that forced retirement is welcomed by some of the elderly; it can provide a graceful means for bowing out of unwanted struggles for jobs and promotions. But that is beside the point. The point is that forced retirement strips elderly individuals of major privileges of economic citizenship, and some of the elderly do not want to relinquish these privileges. This is not only unfair to some elderly individuals, it is not necessarily best for the greater good. A particular individual over the age of 70, whose economic citizenship is rescinded by forced retirement, can have more job-relevant ability than younger individuals whose citizenship is not denied. The societal contributions of the elderly can thus be lost through enforcement of forced retirement policies in which the rule of averages is applied, irrespective of the particular characteristics of elderly individuals.

Often, the injustice of such rulings is not recognized. There have been few legal questionings of laws based on the rule of averages. There is no necessary relation between the appropriateness of a ruling and the quality of the evidence on which the ruling is based. Poor evidence can lead to a correct conclusion. It is possible that although the common sense evidence does not provide a sound basis for rulings that seriously affect the elderly, other evidence—better evidence—does provide such a basis. So we must ask, "Does the scientific evidence support the same kinds of conclusions as are suggested by the evidence of common sense?" The Gillund contribution to this symposium provides an excellent review of that part of the scientific evidence that has accumulated in the behavioral sciences.

Gillund's review indicates that a substantial body of scientific evidence indicates that there are, on the average for many individuals, aging losses in particular intellectual abilities that are important for human adjustment and adaptation. In particular, the evidence indicates aging losses in what Gillund referred to as "processing resources." Processing resources are important parts of fluid intellect, abbreviated Gf (Horn 1985). Gf is expressed in tasks that require reasoning in relatively novel situations and reasoning under conditions in which knowledge of the culture is not sufficient for comprehending relations and drawing proper inferences. Prominent among Gf abilities are capacities for encoding information.

Loss of Gf ability (processing resources) is important whether or not one can compensate for the loss with adroit use of knowledge structure. Knowledge structure is another term for what is widely known (in theory of cognitive abilities) as crystallized or Gc abilities. As Gillund pointed out, the scientific evidence suggests that the Gc (knowledge structure) increases with age in adulthood, at least up to about age 70. In practical terms, this means that the older person has better access to a larger store of knowledge than the younger person. In some cases, the Gc abilities can be applied to the solution of novel reasoning problems such as might seem to depend primarily on Gf. Just how general this kind of substitution of one set of abilities for another might be in "real life" (i.e., outside the restrictions of psychological research) is not known, but it seems likely that it cannot always suffice, that Gc abilities cannot always be applied to compensate for lack of Gf abilities. It seems, too, that Gf reasoning is needed for problem solving that is important in human affairs.

There is, then, some support for the common sense notion that important intellectual abilities decline with age in adulthood and might become notably low after about age 70. It is important to notice, however, that the scientific evidence, not less than the common sense evidence, is based on averages in respect to which there are substantial variations. This can be seen in the results of a recent study of practically all the data in the literature that is both longitudinal and obtained with the Wechsler Adult Intelligence Scales (the WAIS) (McArdle, Aber and Horn 1986).

In longitudinal studies, the same person is measured both at a young age and at an older age. There is systematic attrition in such samples. Aging people of low ability, for whom the decline in abilities tends to be greatest, return less frequently for retesting than do people of high ability. Those of low ability, thus, are underrepresented in longitudinal studies. Other factors produce sample bias in longitudinal studies (Horn and Donaldson 1980). Nevertheless, at a general level, the evidence obtained with longitudinal studies is consistent with the evidence derived from cross-sectional sampling in which the attrition is of a different nature. The conclusions suggested by the longitudinal results are consistent with conclusions derived from the major body of evidence on aging changes in intellectual abilities.

This evidence indicates no stable variation around the averages that define the curves of age changes. The curve of averages for Gc (knowledge structure) at different ages increases throughout the range of adulthood, but the variation around this curve also increases notably throughout this developmental period. This means that some older people score substantially lower than the average of younger people, even when most older people and older people on the average score higher than comparable younger people and younger people on the average. Fair application of the rules of averages would lead to favoring the elderly over the youthful, but the variation around the curve of averages cautions against this when considering particular individuals. Similarly, the curve of averages for Gf (processing resources) indicates aging decline. The variations around the averages at different ages are approximately the same. But here, too, the evidence indicates that some younger people score substantially lower than the average of older people. Variation around the averages indicates the need to consider the competence of the particular individual regardless of that individual's age.

Thus, the scientific evidence, just as the common sense evidence, indicates that rules and laws based on averages are not just and are not sensible when applied to some of the individuals on which the averages are based. This is true even when there is relatively little variation around the averages (although the problems of inappropriate generalization arise less frequently under these conditions).

Overall, scientific evidence illustrates that there is good reason to question the common sense belief that because a particular person has lost his abilities, all people as old as this person or older have lost their abilities. The results indicate that the resource of intellectual power decreases with age when that power is measured in terms of Gf ability for reasoning in *novel problem-solving situations,* but intellectual power increases with age when it is measured in terms of the Gc abilities of knowledge structure.

How should this evidence be used in decisions pertaining to the elderly—in decisions about the allocation of land, labor, and capital for health care for the elderly? I must leave the complexities of this question to economists and other experts, but at a simple level, I suggest that the intellectual resources of the elderly should be used, and health care for the elderly should be allocated roughly in proportion to the elderly's contribution to the common good.

One problem with these suggestions is that, presently, the intellectual resources of the elderly often are not used; in our society, there is considerable inertia to maintain this condition. Therefore, only relatively small allocations of resources of health care for the elderly can be justified on grounds that it is commensurate with the elderly's contributions to the society.

Lack of use of the intellectual (and other) resources of the elderly stems partly from widespread acceptance of the idea that people should retire from work in the later years of adulthood. As mentioned earlier, this idea derives from the belief that intellectual resources of the elderly have been expended.

A resource that is not used is not present in the balancing of compensations. If the intellectual resources of the elderly are not used because the elderly are retired from the work force, then the claim of the elderly for health care resources is very much weakened. As a group, the elderly have accepted forced retirement—indeed some (perhaps many) have welcomed it. The result is that when expenditures must be pruned, health care for the elderly is likely to be regarded as an expendable luxury.

The individual physician, under obligation of his Hippocratic oath, will apply all available resources to the health care of a particular elderly patient. But this same physician will make decisions that limit the available resources for treatment of the elderly if it is believed that the elderly as a group do not contribute notably to the common weal. To the extent that the intellectual resources of the elderly are not used, there will be a decrease in the allocation of health-care resources for their care.

Suzanne Dandoy has raised questions about what might be the basis for rationing preventive health-care practices for the elderly. The elderly make a poor case for deserving this kind of resource if they contribute little to the intellectual work of the society. Acceptance of the belief that the elderly must retire (for whatever reason) leads to this poor case.

If the elderly don't like this state of affairs, it is up to them to change it. In particular, it is up to them to use their intellectual resources to change the prevalent belief that their intellectual resources do not exist. It is up to them to change conditions that force them into unwanted retirement. It is up to them to change—if they want to change—their ideas about the desirability of retirement. Otherwise, they should expect to come up short any time there is rationing of health-care resources.

References

Horn, J. L. 1985. "Remodeling Old Models of Intelligence." In *Handbook of Intelligence*, B. B. Wolman, ed. New York: John Wiley & Sons Inc.

Horn, J. L. and G. Donaldson. 1980. "Cognitive Development in Adulthood." In *Constancy and Change in Human Development*, O. G. Brim and J. Kapan, eds. Cambridge, Mass.: Harvard University Press.

McArdle, J. J., M. S. Aber and J. L. Horn. *Aging and Abilities: A Repeated Measures Meta-analysis of the WAIS* (forthcoming).

4

Age Rationing and the Just Distribution of Health Care: Is There a Duty to Die?

Margaret P. Battin

IN THE FIFTH CENTURY B.C., Euripides addressed "those who patiently endure long illnesses" as follows:

> I hate the men who would prolong their lives
> By foods and drinks and charms of magic art
> Perverting nature's course to keep off death
> They ought, when they no longer serve the land
> To quit this life, and clear the way for youth.[1]

These lines express a view again stirring controversy: that the elderly who are irreversibly ill, whose lives can be continued only with substantial medical support, ought not to be given treatment; instead, their lives should be brought to an end. It should be recognized, as one contemporary political figure is said to have put it, that they "have a duty to die."[2]

Although this controversy achieves a new urgency as pressures for containment of health care costs escalate, the notion is hardly new that there is a time for the ill elderly to die, a time at which they are obligated to bring their lives to an end or allow others to do so. A

This article is reprinted by courtesy of *Ethics*, January 1987 issue. I would like to thank Bruce Landesman, Leslie Francis, Tim Smeeding, Peter Windt, Dan Wikler, Tom Reed, and Virgil Aldrich for their comments on an earlier draft. Some material in this chapter is drawn from an earlier paper "Choosing the Time to Die: The Ethics and Economics of Suicide in Old Age," in *Geriatrics and Ethics: Value Conflicts for the 21st Century*, edited by I. Lawson, S. Spicker, and S. Ingman (Dordrecht: D. Reidel Publishing Co.), forthcoming.

number of conspicuous voices throughout history have advanced such a notion, variously recommending denial of treatment, euthanasia, or socially-assisted "rational" suicide as a means of bringing it about. Plato, for instance, said that the chronically ill or disabled patient ought to refuse medical treatment, and if he cannot return to work, simply die.[3] In Thomas More's *Utopia*, the priests and magistrates are to urge the person who suffers a painful incurable illness "to make the decision not to nourish such a painful disease any longer," and to "deliver himself from the scourge and imprisonment of living or let others release him."[4] Nietzsche claimed that the physician should administer a "fresh dose of disgust," rather than a prescription, to the sick man who "continues to vegetate in a state of cowardly dependence upon doctors" and who thus becomes a "parasite" on society; it is "indecent," he says, "to go on living."[5]

Not only have individual thinkers recommended such practices, but a variety of primitive and historical societies appear to have engaged in them. Although the anthropological data may not be fully reliable, there seems to be evidence of a variety of senicide practices, variously involving abandonment, direct killing, or socially enforced suicide. The Eskimo, for instance, are reported to have practiced suicide in old age "not merely to be rid of a life that is no longer a pleasure, but also to relieve their nearest relations of the trouble they give them."[6] The early Japanese are said to have taken their elderly to a mountaintop to die.[7] Various migratory American Indian tribes abandoned their infirm members by the side of the trail. At least while it was under siege, the Greeks on the island of Ceos required persons reaching the age of sixty-five to commit suicide. Except within the school headed by Hippocrates, Greek physicians apparently made euthanasia or assistance in suicide available to those whose illnesses they could not cure, and there is some evidence that the hemlock was developed for this purpose.[8] Greek and Roman Stoics—most notably Seneca—recommended suicide as the responsible act of the wise man, who ought not assign overly great importance to mere life itself, but rather achieve the disengagement and wisdom required to end his own life at the appropriate time. Of course, not all of these practices have been humane, either in their initial intent or in their final outcome; although the early Nazi euthanasia program known as T4, which practiced active termination of the lives of chronically ill, debilitated, or retarded Aryans, was advertised as a benefit to these persons as well as to the state, it became the training ground for concentration camp personnel.[9] But although practices that range from recommending refusal of medical treatment to encouraging suicide to deliberate, involuntary killing may seem to differ sharply in their ethical characteristics, there is nevertheless an important, central similarity: they are all the practices of societies that communicate to their members that when they reach advanced old age or become irreversibly ill, it is time to die, and that they have an obligation to acquiesce or cooperate in bringing this about. The question to be explored here, in the light of current issues concerning distributive justice in health care, is whether there is any moral warrant at all to this view, and if so, precisely what consequences this would have for the health care of the aged.

The Economics of Health Care for the Aged

In contemporary society, a discomforting set of economic facts brings this issue into prominence. Health care use by the aged constitutes a major component of medical spending, and exacerbates that scarcity of medical resources that generates distributive dilemmas in the first place. People reaching old age, and especially those entering extreme old age, are people for whom late life dependency has or may become a reality, for whom medical care expenses are likely to escalate, and for whom needs for custodial and nursing care will increase. Three out of four deaths of persons of all ages in the United States occur as a result of degenerative diseases, and the proportion is much higher in old age;[10] the multiple infirmities and extended downhill course characteristic of these diseases greatly elevates the need for medical care. People over 65 use medical services at 3.5 times the rate of those below 65.[11] In 1981, the 11 percent of the population over 65 used 39.3 percent of short-stay hospital days, and the 4.4 percent over 75 used 20.7 percent.[12] There are now about six million octogenarians, and the federal government provides an estimated $51 billion in transfers and services to them.[13] People 80 years of age or older consume, on average, 77 percent more medical benefits than those between 65 and 79.[14] Nursing home residents number about 1.5 million, of whom 90 percent are 65 or over, at an average cost of $20,000 per year.[15] Although only 4.7 percent of persons 65 or over are in nursing homes, rates rise with age. About one percent of persons 65–74 are in nursing homes; of those 75–84, seven percent, and of those 85 and over, about 20 percent are in nursing homes on any given day.[16] Even so, institutionalized persons represent a comparatively small fraction of the elderly suffering chronic illnesses and disabilities, and it is estimated that for every nursing home resident, there are two other people with equivalent disabilities in the community.[17] Even if a person maintains functional independence into old age, the risk of becoming frail for a prolonged period is still high: for independent persons between 65 and 69, one study found, total life expectancy was 16.5 years, but "active life expectancy," or the portion of the remaining years that were characterized by independence, was only ten years, and the remaining 6.5 years were characterized by major functional impairment. Furthermore, this risk increases with age: persons who were independent at 85 were likely to spend 60 percent of their remaining 7.3 years requiring assistance.[18] Expenditures are particularly large for those who are about to die: for instance, for Medicare enrollees in 1976, the average reimbursement for those in their last year of life was 6.2 times as large as for those who survived at least two years, and although those who died comprised only 5.9 percent of Medicare enrollees, they accounted for 27.9 percent of program expenditures.[19] Thirty percent of all expenses of decedents occurred in the last 30 days of life, 46 percent in the last 60 days, and 77 percent in the last six months of life.[20] While this figure is not confined to deaths among the elderly, a 1983 survey of cancer deaths for Blue Cross/Blue Shield predicted that the average American who died of cancer in that year would incur more than $22,000 of illness-related expenses during the final year of life.[21]

Clearly, contemporary analogues of the practices of the historical and primitive societies mentioned above, ranging from refusal or denial of treatment to outright senicide and societally mandated suicide, would have pronounced impact upon the health care resources available for other persons in society. It is this that gives rise to the painful distributive question to be examined here. If scarcity precludes granting all persons within society all the care they need for all medical conditions that might arise, some persons or some conditions must be reduced or excluded from care. But if so, it is often held, those excluded should be the elderly ill: after all, the medical conditions from which they suffer are often extraordinarily expensive to treat; the prognosis, as age increases, is increasingly poor; and in any case, they have already lived full life spans and had claim to a fair share of societal resources. It is this view, or constellation of views, that seems to underlie and motivate practices suggesting that there is a time for the elderly to die.

Justice and Age Rationing

If societal resources are insufficient to provide all the health care all persons in all medical conditions need, some sort of limiting distributive practice will of necessity emerge. Several recent writers have argued that rather than let the market control the distribution of health care, a rationally defended rationing policy can be developed under accepted principles of justice, and that this policy will justify rationing by age: old people should be the first to be excluded from medical care. However, assuming the underlying formal principle of justice to require that like cases and groups be treated alike, it is by no means initially clear that plausible material principles of justice will differentiate the elderly from other claimants for care. For instance, if an individual's claim to care were taken to be a function of the contributions society may expect as a return on its investment in him, this might seem to support age rationing, disfavoring those no longer capable of making contributions; but of course the elderly have already made contributions, contributions that are, in fact, more secure than the potential contributions of the young. Alternatively, it might be argued that the elderly have greater claims to care in virtue of their greater vulnerability, in virtue of the respect owed elders, or in virtue of the intrinsic value of old age. This sort of discussion, characteristic of many analyses of distributive justice, involves identifying the possible desert bases of claims to health care, and then considering whether the elderly can satisfy these conditions as well as other age groups. If they can (which I think likely), policies that restrict the access of the elderly to health care must be seen as the product of simple age bias.

But an influential conceptual observation has been made by Norman Daniels.[22] Most analyses of distributive justice, Daniels observes, assume that the elderly constitute one among a variety of age groups, including infants, adolescents, and the middle-aged, all of whom compete for scarce resources in health care. But this, in Daniels' view, is misleading; the elderly should be viewed as the same persons at a later stage of their lives. The mistake lies in considering distributive problems as problems in allocating resources among competing groups and among competing individuals, when they are more correctly understood as problems of allocating resources throughout the duration of lives. Given this conceptual shift, Daniels then employs Rawlsian strategies to determine just allocations of care. He considers what distributive policies prudential savers—the rational, self-interest-maximizing parties of the Rawlsian original position— would adopt if, unable to know their own medical conditions, genetic predispositions, physical susceptibilities, environmental situations, health maintenance habits, or ages, they must decide in advance on a spending plan budgeting a fixed amount of medical care across their whole lives. He quite plausibly conjectures that prudential savers behind the veil of ignorance in this original position would choose, where scarcity obtains, to allocate a greater amount of resources to care and treatment required for conditions that occur earlier in life, from infancy through middle age, but not to underwrite treatment that would prolong life beyond its normal span. By freeing resources that might otherwise have been devoted to prolonging the lives of the elderly, so that they are used instead to treat diseases that cause death or disability earlier in life, such a policy would maximize one's chances of receiving a reasonable amount of life within the normal species-typical, age-relative opportunity range. (Presumably, such a policy would not allocate extensive care to severely defective neonates, catastrophically and irreversibly damaged accident victims, or other persons whose medical prognoses are so dismal that the prospect of achieving even remotely normal species-typical, age-relative opportunity is extremely poor. Thus, savings resulting from rationing care to the elderly would not be entirely consumed in treating the worst-off newborns or others in similarly hopeless circumstances, and the "black hole" problem would be avoided.) If this is a policy upon which prudential savers would agree, Daniels holds, it will show that—at least under scarcity conditions against a background of just institutions—age-rationing is morally warranted for making allocations of health care.

But this leaves unanswered a crucial issue of application. If, in a situation of scarcity, a rationally defended rationing policy for health care resources is more just than market control, and if the most just form of rationing for health care is rationing by age, this still does not determine what policies and practices for putting age-rationing into effect are themselves just. Arguments for rationing are always morally incomplete without attention to the crucial details of precisely how such policies are to be given effect, since intolerable features of such policies may force reconsideration of the rationing strategy from the start. Thus, employing Daniels's Rawlsian strategy, it is necessary to consider what age-rationing policies rational self-interest maximizers in the original position would accept.

Whatever merits it may have as an application of the Rawlsian conception of justice, Daniels's strategy is intuitively attractive for assessing the moral justifiability of age-rationing in health care. This is because those of us considering this issue—who would be prepared to develop policy requirements on the basis of these considerations and who would be governed by whatever policies might be devised— are effectively behind the "veil of ignorance" with respect to the specific events of our own aging and death. While Rawls claims that we can enter the original position any time simply by reasoning for principles of justice in accordance with the appropriate restrictions on not taking into account one's own specific interests,[23] such self-restriction is hardly necessary: when considering issues of justice with respect to aging and death, we are already there. It is, of course, true that most persons who are reasonably familiar with background medical and genetic information and who have some knowledge of their own ancestry, previous health history, and health maintenance habits are not completely ignorant of the probable circumstances of their own aging and death. Yet they are able to eliminate with certainty only a very few types and causes of death (e.g., specific hereditary diseases for which one is not at risk), and to assign rough probabilities to the likelihood of contracting the major killer diseases. Even those with early symptoms of a disease syndrome cannot be sure that some other fatal condition will not intervene. What they are not able to do is prospectively identify with certainty the actual cause of their own deaths or the precise events of a future terminal course. By and large, persons still in a position to consider the issue of health care age-rationing for the elderly and to develop policy responses do not yet know when or how they will age and die. But we are all in this position, and we find ourselves obliged to evaluate policies and applications of age-rationing practices without knowing how they will affect our own interests when the time comes. Yet despite the fact that we thus replicate the Rawlsian original position quite naturally, our reluctance to look squarely at death and its often unpleasant circumstances may undermine both the rationality and the justice of the death-related policies we adopt.

If the Rawls/Daniels strategy is employed, then, possible practices and policies for effecting age-rationing, including denial or refusal of treatment, senicide, euthanasia, and socially mandated "rational" suicide, are to be assessed in terms of whether rational self-interest maximizers behind the veil of ignorance would agree to accept such policies or not. However, despite the analogy between the lack of specific knowledge characteristic of parties to the original position and the lack of specific knowledge characteristic of ordinary persons who have not yet reached old age or death, what rational self-interest maximizers in the original position would agree to cannot be determined simply by inspecting the age and death-related choices of ordinary persons now. This is because the kinds of choices we ordinary persons make are very heavily determined by social expectation and custom, legal and religious restrictions, paternalistic practices in medicine, financial limitations, and so on. Furthermore, as ordinary persons, we may fail both to realize what our own self-interests actually are and to choose the most efficient means of satisfying them. Consequently, it is necessary to consider—as far as possible independently of cultural constraints—what policies for putting age-rationing into practice the hypothetical rational, self-interest-maximizing persons in the original position would accept, given that they have antecedently consented to policies assigning enhanced care to the early and middle years, but reducing care to the aged. Parties to the original position have disenfranchised themselves, so to speak; but it remains to be seen what form they would agree this disenfranchisement should take.

Age-Rationing by Denial of Treatment

Although in order to enhance health care available to younger and middle-aged people and thus maximize the possibility of each person's reaching a normal life span at all, parties to the original position will have already agreed to ration health care to the elderly, they must be assumed to have enough general information to see what the consequences of this antecedent agreement will be. First, under an appropriately thin veil of ignorance, they will know that a given measure of health care is not equally effective at all age ranges, but much more effective in younger years, much less effective in old age. Because old persons typically have more complex medical problems, compounded by a decline in the function of many organs and by reduced capacities for healing and homeostasis, tradeoffs between earlier and later years cannot be made on a one-to-one basis: by and large, a unit of medical care consumed late in life will have much less effect in preserving life and maintaining normal species-typical function than a unit of medical care consumed at a younger age. It is this that will have, in part, induced the rational self-interest maximizers of the original position to consent to an age-rationing policy in the first place; but it will also influence how they choose to put an age-rationing policy into effect. Once the multiple infirmities of old age begin to erode an individual's functioning, comparatively larger amounts of health care are likely to be required to raise it again. Therapy that can successfully maintain comfort, or restore functioning, or preserve life may be very much more expensive in older patients, if indeed successful treatment is possible at all.

Parties to the original position will also know that under a rationing scheme it will be necessary, given their antecedent distributive decision, to restrict or eliminate most of the comparatively elaborate kinds of care. Presumably, if care is to be denied, it will be the highest-cost, least-gain varieties of care, including care that does not directly serve to maintain life. Of course, "cheap treatment" such as common antibiotics could be retained for elderly patients, since these are low-cost and, given their potential for saving life, high-gain; but expensive diagnostic procedures and therapies like CAT scans, NMR, dialysis, organ transplants, hip replacements, hydrotherapy, respiratory support, total parenteral nutrition, individualized physical therapy, vascular grafting, major surgery, and high-tech procedures generally would be ruled out.[24] Hospitalization, and the nearly equal expensive inpatient hospice care, might not be permitted, except perhaps briefly; sustained nursing home care (at $20,000 a year) would no doubt also be excluded. When the elderly person over an appropriate age ceiling or exceeding a predetermined level of deterioration begins to show symptoms of a condition more serious than a transitory, easily cured illness, he would simply be considered ineligible for treatment. "I'm sorry, Mr. Smith," we can expect the physician to say, "there is nothing more we can do."

Knowing these things, parties to the original position can then assess the impact of age rationing by denial of treatment. While they will know that age rationing of some of the more expensive, elaborate treatment modalities, like renal dialysis and organ transplantation, is now prevalent in Britain,[25] and is to an uneven extent also evident in the United States,[26] they will also understand that under the general age rationing policy they have agreed to, the frequency and finality of such denials of treatment would be much more severe. Although allocations to the elderly would, of course, be a fluctuating function of scarcity in health care resources as a whole, it is probably fair to estimate that were the degree of scarcity approximately equivalent to what it is now, a just distribution of health care would demand that a very large proportion of all health care expenses now devoted to the elderly be reassigned to younger age groups. The elderly now use nearly one-third of all health care.[27] Were these resources reassigned to the younger and middle-aged groups, the probability would dramatically increase that all, or virtually all, these persons (except the worst-off newborns and those catastrophically injured or killed outright in accidents, homicide, or suicide) would not only reach a normal life span, but reach it in reasonably good health. Although the temporary life expectancy (or average number of years a group of persons at the beginning of an age interval will live during that age interval) is already very high, especially for the intervals 0–20 and 20–45,[28] it is still the case that a sizeable number of people do not reach a normal life span, or reach it only in poor health.[29] Reallocation of substantial health care resources would do a great deal to change this, particularly if the transfers were used for preventive medicine and support programs, such as prenatal nutrition and lifestyle change, as well as direct assaults on specific diseases. But to achieve this effect, if the degree of overall scarcity of medical resources could not be altered, a substantial portion of the care now given the elderly would have to be withdrawn. At most, perhaps, minimal home hospice care and inexpensive pain relief could be routinely granted, together with some superficial care in transient acute illness not related to chronic conditions or interdependent diseases. But treatment for the elderly could not be escalated very much beyond this point if, within a fixed degree of scarcity, a just distribution of resources were still to be achieved: if only a significantly lesser portion of the care now devoted to the elderly were reassigned to younger age groups, there would be no substantial redistributive achievement and no significant increase in the prospects for persons generally for reaching a normal life span. Minimal and erratic age-rationing of the sort now practiced in the United States would accomplish virtually no redistributive goal at all.

In some cases, to deny the elderly treatment beyond minimal home hospice care and inexpensive pain relief would simply result in earlier deaths. This would, presumably, be the case in many sorts of acute conditions—heart attacks or sudden-onset renal failure, for instance—where emergency medical intervention is clearly lifesaving. But, especially in old age, such starkly life vs. death episodes are less likely to occur in isolation; it is much more likely that an elderly person will already suffer from a number of related or unrelated chronic conditions, each of which could be relieved, at least to some degree, by treatment, but which together make a fairly substantial and expensive list of complaints. Almost half the persons age 65 or older suffer from chronic conditions,[30] of which the most frequently reported for the noninstitutionalized elderly are arthritis, vision and hearing impairments, heart conditions, and hypertension.[31] The elderly over 85 in the community average 3.5 important disabilities per person, and those who are hospitalized 6.[32] Some of these chronic conditions are extremely common, like visual impairment, arthritis, and loss of hearing, but they are not always inexpensive to treat. Many of the conditions associated with increasing age, like Alzheimer's, certain types of arthritis and cancers, osteoporosis, or stroke, may require extended medical, nursing, or rehabilitative care. But extended, substantial medical, nursing, and rehabilitative care is expensive; consequently, these are precisely the conditions in which, in a just health care system under conditions of scarcity, the elderly would be denied care.

Clearly, even hypothetical parties to the original position, under an appropriately thin veil of ignorance, will be dismayed by the consequences of the initial distributive decision they have made. Total hip replacements, for instance, could no longer be offered the elderly; but it will be evident that there is a substantial difference in the character of life for an elderly person who remains ambulatory and one no longer able to walk. It will be evident, too, that the person who needs, but does not receive, a pacemaker or a coronary bypass may lead a very restricted life, seriously limited in his activities; and that life with renal failure, or cardiac arrhythmias, or pulmonary insufficiency can be restrictive, painful, or frightening. Indeed, what may be most dismaying to those peering through this thin veil of ignorance is that elderly persons who are not allocated treatment do not simply die; rather, they suffer their illness and disabilities without adequate aid. Even symptom control in conditions like cancer, if not simply obliterative of consciousness, can be quite expensive, since effective relief may require constant titration and monitoring; if so, it too would presumably be ruled out. Worse still, common antibiotics and the few other kinds of cheap treatment that would still be available may simply serve to prolong this period of decline, not to reduce its discomforts, while labor-intensive care that might make it tolerable— like physical therapy or psychiatric support and counseling—would also be ruled out. To deny treatment does not always simply bring about earlier deaths that maximal care would postpone; denial of treatment also means denial of expensive palliative measures, both physical and psychological, which maximal care would permit at whatever age death occurs.

Nor can it be supposed that to deny care to the elderly is to simply allow them to die as their fathers and forefathers did; to deny care now is to subject persons to a medically new situation. Not only has it been comparatively unlikely, until quite recently, that a person would reach old age at all (in the United States, life expectancy at birth in 1900 was only 47.3 years, compared to 74.5 in 1982[33]), but in the past, most deaths were caused by parasitic and infectious diseases, many of which were rapidly fatal. Modern sanitation, inoculation, and antibiotic therapy have changed that, and for the first time, the specter of old age as a constellation of various sublethal but severely limiting and discomforting conditions has become the norm. Hence, any notion that denial of treatment to the elderly will simply allow a return to the more "natural" modes of death enjoyed by earlier, simpler generations is a dangerously romanticized misconception. To ration health care by denial of treatment is not simply to abandon the patient to death, but often to abandon him to a prolonged period of morbidity, only later followed by death.

But, of course, this is a prospect that the rational self-interest maximizer, behind the veil of ignorance about whether he himself will succumb quickly in an acute crisis or be consigned without substantial medical assistance to a long-term decline, will be concerned to protect against. Parties to the original position will thus find many reasons to reject policies that ration health care by denying treatment to the aged; the question for them will be whether they can devise better alternative methods.

Squaring the Curve

Since the publication in 1980 of James Fries's provocative article on the compression of morbidity,[34] there has been a good deal of discussion of the end-of-life morbidity characteristic of old age. Although the average life span in the United States has increased more than 26 years between 1900 and the present, Fries points out, the maximum life span has not increased; there is no greater percentage of centenarians, for instance, and there are no documented cases of survival, he claims, beyond 114 years. The result is an increasingly "rectangularized" mortality curve, as more and more people reach old age but the maximum old age is not extended. Furthermore, since this rectangularization results from postponement of the onset of chronic illness, it means an increasingly rectangularized morbidity curve as well. On this basis, Fries optimistically predicts that the number of extremely old persons will not increase, that the average period of diminished physical vigor or senescence will decrease, that chronic disease will occupy a smaller proportion of the typical life span, and that the need for medical care in late life will decrease. Good health, in short, will extend closer and closer to the ideal average life span of about 85, but life will not be extended much beyond this point.

Fries's conclusions about "squaring the curve," as it is often called, have been vigorously disputed by Schneider and Brody,[35] among others. They see no evidence of declining morbidity and disability in any age group, particularly those just prior to old age, but they do observe that increasing numbers of people are reaching advanced ages, and point out that this fast-growing segment of the population is the one most vulnerable to chronic disease. While some writers set the biologic limit to the human life span at about 100, much higher

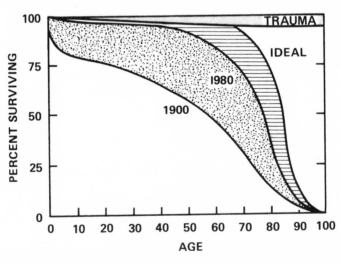

Figure 4.1. Fries Increasingly Rectangular Survival Curve. About 80% (stippled areas) of the difference between the 1900 curve and the ideal curve (stippled area plus hatched area) had been eliminated by 1980. Trauma is now the dominant cause of death in early life. (From Fries, *op. cit.*, p. 131, fig. 2.) Reprinted by courtesy of The New England Journalof Medicine.

than Fries's original estimate of 85, others believe that there is no such limit. In either case, most of these comparatively pessimistic writers fear that a large increase in the number of individuals who reach old age will mean a large increase in persons who spend long proportions of their lives afflicted with chronic disease. Advances in medicine will, they believe, prolong old age rather than delay its onset.

Clearly this issue is one with enormous consequences for health care planning. But it has been debated as an empirical issue only; nowhere has it been recognized that the empirical question cloaks a central moral issue as well. What is crucial to note is that both the optimist and pessimist parties to this dispute agree, or tacitly agree, on one thing: that a squared morbidity curve is a desirable thing. This is by no means surprising: the squared curve represents a situation in which life is, as Fries puts it, "physically, emotionally, and intellectually vigorous until just before its close."[36] Death without illness, or without sustained, long-term illness, rational self-interest maximizers would surely agree, is a desirable thing. But if this is so, the empirical disagreement between the optimists and the pessimists grows irrelevant. For, regardless of whether changes in lifestyle or improvements in medical care would naturally flatten or square the mortality and morbidity curves, these curves can also be deliberately altered by other distributive and policy-based interventions as well—including those that implement age-rationing schemes.

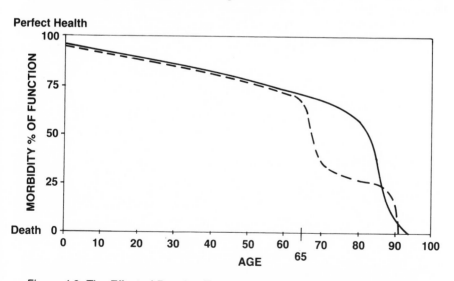

Figure 4.2. The Effect of Denying Treatment in Old Age. The solid line shows the morbidity curve characteristic for a representative individual where treatment is supplied; the dashed line shows the conjectural morbidity curve where treatment is denied after age 65 in sublethal chronic conditions.

As seen in the previous section, rationing that proceeds by denial of treatment may have the effect of not only hastening both the onset and termination of the drop-off or downhill slope of the morbidity curve—patients become impaired earlier and die sooner—but, in many cases, flattening this downslope: the period of senescence, or chronic old-age disability, occupies a longer proportion of life, since it is endured without treatment. The morally significant feature of rationing policies that deny treatment is not simply their effect on mortality rates, but their effect on the ways in which people die.

But the curve can also be artificially squared—by deliberately bringing about death before the onset of serious morbidity, while the quality of life remains comparatively high. This too means that the onset and termination of the drop-off slope are both earlier—the termination a good deal earlier—but the slope itself is now perpendicular, not gradual, and life is terminated with only incipient decline. This is precisely the effect of the primitive and historical practices mentioned earlier: senicide, euthanasia, and socially mandated "rational" suicide, at least where they are practiced early in the downhill course of a long-term degenerative disease. The squared curve will be produced, of course, by denial of treatment in sudden-onset life-threatening conditions, but these are much less characteristic of old age, and the more frequent effect of denying treatment is a flattened,

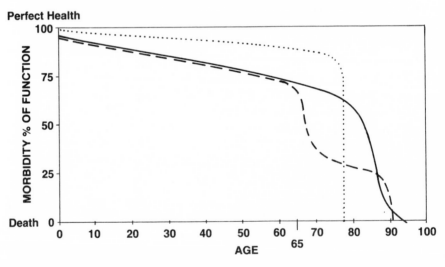

Figure 4.3. Morbidity Curve of Direct-Termination Practices. Solid line shows morbidity curve in old age with treatment, dashed line without treatment, and dotted line shows conjectural morbidity curves in direct-termination practices such as senicide, early euthanasia, and culturally mandated "rational" suicide.

prolonged decline. Practices that guarantee a squared curve, on the other hand, involve direct killing, and, in particular, killing of persons whose quality of life is still comparatively high; nevertheless, these practices do achieve what is agreed by all to be desirable, namely, death without prior sustained, long-term disease.

Under the assumptions employed here, parties to the original position have antecedently contracted for age-rationing policies, even though these will have the effect of reducing the remaining length of life for those who reach old age. In virtue of this initial agreement, these parties are now also in a position to agree upon the sorts of policies by means of which this age rationing will be put into effect. Hence, they must choose between treatment-denying policies and those that impose death; constrained by their earlier decision in favor of age rationing, they no longer have the option of choosing policies that allocate extensive resources to the elderly and thus make possible the extension of life. To put it in the familiar terms of bioethics, they must choose between policies that involve "killing" and those that involve "allowing to die," and their agreement will serve to identify which policy is more just.

For the most part, the age-rationing practices now followed in Britain and the United States, as well as elsewhere, involve denial of treatment, for instance in the form of age ceilings for organ transplants, renal dialysis, or joint replacement. But I wish to argue that rational self-interest maximizers in the original position would prefer the direct-killing practices that are the contemporary analogues of the historical and primitive practices of senicide, early euthanasia, and culturally-encouraged suicide to those that involve allowing to die. Parties to the original position, after all, are fully informed about the possible societal consequences of their choices (except about the impact on themselves) and are not hesitant, as rational persons, to look the circumstances of death squarely in the face. There are, I think, two principal reasons why they would agree on direct-termination policies involving the causing of death, that is, on "squaring the curve."

Avoidance of Suffering

Except for persons who believe, on religious or other grounds, that suffering is of intrinsic merit or is of extrinsic value in attaining salvation or some other valued goal, rational persons eager to maximize their self-interests seek to avoid discomfort, disability, and pain. Of course, a good deal of suffering may willingly be endured by those who hope to survive a critical episode and return to a more normal condition of life; but terminal suffering known to be terminal is not prized. In medical situations where the prognosis is uncertain and sophisticated techniques are employed to support survival, the risk of suffering is one the rational person may well wish to take, since the odds of survival may be either unknown or large enough to make it worth the risk. But under an age-rationing system that proceeds by denial of treatment, medical support will be minimal, and hence comparatively ineffective in supporting survival; the chance of survival of an episode of illness is thereby drastically reduced. Thus, the possible gains to be achieved by enduring suffering disappear. Willingness to endure suffering may be a prudent, self-interest favoring posture in a medical climate in which support is provided—even if that support is erratic or the chance of success is unknown—but it is not a prudent posture where age rationing precludes nearly all such support across the board.

Maximization of Life

Parties to the original position will also give preference to a policy that involves an overall distributive gain, benefitting all, but giving the greatest benefit to the least advantaged. Since the allocation of resources may affect the overall total of resources available, they will prefer policies that maximize resources in a just distribution, and it is this that "squaring the curve" would accomplish. Of course, individuals surveying the possibility of policies that permit or require the direct termination of the existence of human beings may believe that their lives are to be sacrificed in the interests of other, younger people, and were this the case, they would rightly resist this sort of utilitarian tradeoff. But individuals who view these prospective policies in this way make a fundamental error: they view the effects of these policies from their own immediate perspective only, and fail to see the larger impact these policies have. Quite the contrary, the overall effect of direct-termination policies is to *maximize* the preservation of life, not reduce it. This is a function of the fact, as pointed out earlier, that medical care is less efficient in old age, more efficient at younger ages, and that a unit of medical care consumed late in life will have much less effect in preserving life and maintaining normal species-typical function than a unit of medical care consumed at a younger age. The effect of rationing policies that allocate care away from elderly persons to younger ones is to increase the effectiveness of these resources, and thus greatly increase the chances for younger persons to reach a normal life span. Of course, since mortality in the 0–20 and 20–45 age ranges is already quite low, the increase in temporary life expectancy will be greatest for those 45–65; but, it must be remembered, the veil of ignorance for those in the original position excludes all but the vaguest knowledge of likelihoods of their own positions,[37] and *any* possibly preventable mortality or morbidity in these younger age ranges will constitute a situation rational self-interest maximizers will work to avoid.

Furthermore, and for the same reasons of efficiency, the reallocation decreases by a much smaller amount the chances for older persons to live beyond a normal life span, since after all those chances were never very great. For example, ten units of medical care given to a 92-year-old man with multiple chronic conditions might make it possible for him to live an additional two years, but ten units of care given to an 8-year-old girl in an acute episode might make it possible for her to live a normal life span, or about 64 additional years. The mistake the disgruntled elderly individual facing a rationing-mandated death makes is in failing to calculate not only the immediate loss he faces, but the benefit he has already gained from policies that have enhanced his chances of reaching his current age: his temporary life expectancy in the ranges 0–20, 20–45, and 45–65 will have been much elevated, even though his total life expectancy may decline. The less the care provided at the end of life, and hence the greater amount of transfer to earlier ages, the greater his gain in life prospects will have been. (Of course, this effect could not be achieved in the first generation of the implementation of such policies.) Furthermore, direct-termination policies are more effective in maximizing overall gains in life saved than denial-of-treatment policies. Since denial-of-treatment practices still always involve some costs as persons with multiple conditions in interrelated degenerative diseases are granted minimal hospice and palliative care during their downhill courses, the proportion of savings is smaller, and less is transferred to earlier age groups.

Consequently, the disgruntled individual also makes a second mistake: he fails to see that because direct termination rather than denial of treatment maximizes the amount of transfer to younger age groups, such a policy will have maximized his own chances (except in the first generation) not just of reaching old age, but of entering it with fewer chronic, preexisting conditions. Furthermore, this policy will have done the same for all other persons as well. But as the number of persons entering old age with chronic conditions decreases, the normal life span will tend to increase (at least to any natural limit there may be), and with it, the chances of any individual's reaching this mark. The long-term effect of such policies— despite the fact that they involve deliberately causing death in people who might continue to live—is to gradually increase the normal life span by delaying the onset of seriously debilitating and eventually fatal disease.

The rational person in the original position, then, who counts among his self-interests both the avoidance of suffering and the preservation of his life, will correctly see that social policies providing for the direct termination of his life at the onset of substantial morbidity in old age will more greatly enhance his prospects in satisfying these self-interests than any alternative open in a scarcity situation. After all, as a party to the original position, he has no knowledge of his own medical condition or age at any given time. Of course, if there were no benefits to older as well as younger persons from this reallocation, but rather merely the sacrifice of the interests of some people for those of others, parties to the original position could not agree to such policies; but this is not the case. Since such policies do provide benefits for all, and indeed the greatest benefits for the least advantaged (i.e., those who would otherwise die young), they will receive the agreement of all rational persons in the original position. This agreement, then, provides the basis for counting such policies just.

Attitudes Toward Direct-Termination Age Rationing

But of course, the rational self-interest maximizer in the original position can consent only to policies that are psychologically benign, and that do not impose lifelong anguish or fear; this is because parties to the original position are rational in the sense that they will not enter into agreements they know they cannot keep, or can do so only with great difficulty.[38] Age-rationing policies that involve direct killing of the elderly may seem to invite just such anguish, as one cowers a lifetime in fear of being brutally extinguished by an unscrupulous physician or the naked power of the state. Certainly some of the primitive and historical policies mentioned earlier have engendered just this sort of fear; the early Nazi "euthanasia" program, although reserved for Aryans and initially performed with relatives' consent, comes to mind.

Nevertheless, whether death in old age is feared or welcomed is very much a product of social beliefs and expectations, and these not only undergo spontaneous transformations, but can be quite readily altered and engineered.[39] Transformations in social practices in earlier historical periods make it evident that beliefs about whether there is such a thing as a time to die can change; transformation can be equally well imagined in the present. Aristotle's dictum notwithstanding, whether death is believed to be the worst of evils, or whether some circumstances—extreme incapacitation, inability to communicate, or continuous pain—are believed to be worse than death is much influenced by the surrounding society. Mary Rose

Barrington speculates about an attitudinal change that, in the contemporary cost-conscious climate, seems an increasingly real possibility: "What if," she writes, "a time came when, no longer able to look after oneself, the decision to live on for the maximum number of years were considered a mark of heedless egoism? What if it were to be thought that *dulce et decorum est pro familia mori?*"[40]

Many sorts of prevailing social expectations serving the interests of society at large, and hence the long-term interests of individuals, are readily cooperated with, even at some immediate and direct cost to the individuals involved: for example, expectations about getting married, pursuing careers, supporting children, and so on. All of these involve a good deal of societal and institutional support. Marriage is encouraged, in part, by elaborate ceremonies and religious services; universities and technical training schools provide not only employment skills but socialize students to want to pursue careers; the support of children is enforced not only by legal penalties for failure to do so, but by extremely strong social sanctions. It is not at all difficult to imagine the development of social expectations that there is a time to die, or, indeed, that it is a matter of virtue or obligation to choose to die.[41] To be effective, these expectations would presumably be coupled with supportive social practices—for instance, predeath counseling, physician assistance in providing the actual means of inducing death, or ceremonial recognition from such institutions as churches. Clearly, societal expectations concerning the time to die need not be dysphoric or condemn the members of an age-rationing society to lifetimes of anguish or fear. Indeed, Daniels suggests that a view very like this characterized Aleut society:

> The elderly, or the enfeebled elderly, are sent off to die, sparing the rest of the community from the burden of sustaining them. From descriptions of the practice, the elderly quite willingly accept this fate, and it is fair that they should.[42]

Nor need direct-termination rationing policies be viewed as a violation of rights. In an age-rationing society, there is no *right* to live maximally on, nor to receive the necessary medical care. Of course, an individual may have rights to many sorts of things even in a society that rations by age—for instance, a right to termination procedures that are dignified and humane. A person will also have rights to freedom from abuse (to be discussed in the next section). And it will also be the case that younger persons have rights to medical care and the prolongation of life. Consequently, direct-termination age-rationing policies, fairly applied, would not violate that Rawlsian principle of justice that stipulates that each person has an equal right to basic rights and liberties compatible with equal rights and liberties for all, since each person will have had an equal right to medical prolongation of life and equal liberty to live in his younger and middle years, and each person will be equally subject to the expectation that his life will come to an end before sustained terminal morbidity sets in. This policy does not entail that elderly people no longer have rights; they continue to enjoy the rights of persons in society, but the right to extensive medical continuation of their lives is not among them.

The Issue of Abuse

Not only would rational self-interest maximizers in the original position require that any direct-termination rationing policies adopted not be dysphoric in their application nor violate rights, but they will also require that these policies not invite abuse. To abuse a policy includes not only using it to cause harm to individuals, but to alter the practices it permits in such a way as to render the policy itself inherently unstable. Needless to say, virtually any policy can be abused; but some policies invite abuse in a much stronger way, and policies permitting or requiring direct killing may seem to make the strongest possible invitation of all. The issue, then, is whether parties to the original position could devise direct-termination policies that resist abuse or provide adequate protection against it.

Direct-termination age-rationing policies would need to incorporate at least three features as protections against abuse. Without these features, rational self-interest maximizers in the original position could not consent to them.

Preservation of Choice

First, compliance with direct-termination policies would need to be experienced as essentially voluntary at the level of individual choice. This does not mean that individual choice would not be shaped by more general social expectations, but the individual could not be coerced, either legally or socially, into ending his life. Any individual who chose to resist the social expectation that it is time to die, and hence, to endure the disenfranchisement from treatment that would be his lot, would have to be guaranteed the freedom to do so. Hence, in such a world, it could not be said that the ill, elderly individual has a "duty to die"; what he has is a duty to refrain from further use of medical resources. He may then think it prudent to avail himself of the support in direct, painless termination of his life that such a society would offer, instead of finding himself abandoned to die without substantial medical help; but, of course, conceptions of prudence may vary from one individual to another. Indeed, if social acceptance of direct-termination policies were widespread enough to yield sufficient redistributive savings, this would perhaps permit giving those few persons who chose to tough it out additional medical care; this would underscore the voluntary nature of response to a direct-termination social expectation. Preservation of choice is crucial because state or societal coercion not only causes harm but invites rebellion; it is inherently unstable. Yet, the justice of age-rationing in the first place depends on stable enough functioning of the scheme so that the distributive gains in overall life prospects are actually realized, and a scheme that is clearly unstable enough to make such redistributive effects impossible cannot be said to be just.

Rejection of Fixed Time of Death

Second, the timing of direct-termination rationing policies must be based on expected time before death, not on a fixed cutoff age such as 65 (as on the Greek island of Ceos), 72 (the approximate average life expectancy), or 85 (Fries's conjecture)—or, for that matter, any other fixed age. This is because the underlying purpose of rationing is to enhance the length of life span for all members of society; although it will most greatly benefit those who would otherwise die earliest, it must also benefit the elderly as well. The central mechanism of redistributive age rationing is reallocation of treatment from older years to younger ones, where treatment is more efficacious and where the prospects of a longer life span are enhanced for all, especially for those whose life spans would otherwise be quite short. But if a fixed age cutoff point for the elderly were selected, whereby persons below that cutoff receive full treatment and persons above it were expected to end their lives, the original purpose of rationing would be undermined. Clearly, the use of a fixed-age cutoff point would be extraordinarily inefficient, since it would allocate some resources to persons on a clearly terminal course, where the possibility of extension of life is small, and it would also exterminate life where there was no medical treatment required to sustain it. It is not old age itself that is medically expensive; it is the last month, six months, or year or two of life. Variations in costs and efficacy of treatment are not so much a function of time since birth, but time to death.[43] Many octogenarians are vigorously healthy; so are some people in their nineties and beyond. On the other hand, dying can be expensive and medical efforts futile even for those whose ages are not advanced. Still more importantly, avoidance of a fixed-age cutoff point protects the health care system from political encroachments, particularly those that seek cost containment or other political objectives by adjusting the cutoff age downward.

Consequently, parties to the original position would not favor a fixed-age rationing policy, but rather one which, depending on the degree of scarcity, encouraged direct termination via senicide, early euthanasia, or rational suicide only during the last month, half-year, or year of life. Of course, the precise ante-mortem period can be identified with certainly only retrospectively. However, even this does not constitute a fully effective counterargument, since it is usually possible for the experienced physician to recognize, with at least a fair degree of accuracy, the onset of what is likely to be a downhill course ending in death—especially in an elderly patient. Nevertheless, even if such predictions are sometimes inaccurate, the rational self-interest maximizer will still prefer reliance on them in order to maximize his opportunities for continuing life and normal functioning, something that would be jeopardized much more severely by a rigid age cutoff.

Furthermore, since some declines are comparatively rapid, even if not instantaneous, and some prolonged, parties to the original position will seek to maximize their overall opportunities not by agreeing to a policy in which a fixed amount of time at the end of life is held ineligible for care and in which direct termination may be practiced, but by supporting a policy in which disenfranchisement begins only at the onset of profound illness or irremediable chronic disease. After all, the precise duration of a downhill course can rarely be predicted with accuracy, although it can typically be accurately predicted that the course will indeed be downhill. Consequently, parties to the original position will consent to policies that impose disenfranchisement not long after the diagnosis and onset of symptoms of an eventually terminal disease, or at least long enough after the onset to confirm the diagnosis and for the need for medical care to have become pronounced. Hence, the curve would, in fact, never be perfectly squared, and individuals would not have their lives discontinued while they remained in full health, but the timing of disenfranchisement from care and the expectation that it is "time to die" would fall just after the onset of a characteristic downhill course. Just how far down this slope the cutoff point might come would be a function, of course, of the scarcity situation itself, but also of individual, voluntary choices mentioned above.

Public Awareness

Third, it is crucial that not only parties to the original position, but actual persons affected by such policies both know the policies and understand the rationale for them; secretive or propagandistic policies cannot be rationally chosen, nor can ill-founded ones. It is crucial for the stability and, hence, justice of "time to die" policies that persons affected by them understand their own distributive gain; without this understanding, they will remain disgruntled individuals who see only their own loss. But individuals who see only their own losses under a policy constitute a force for change; this renders the policy itself unstable, and an unstable policy cannot operate to produce a just distribution. It is crucial that the man-in-the-street who reaches old age understands that the very fact that he has been able to do so is, in part, the product of his cooperation with policies that have him accept the claim that it is time to die when serious morbidity sets in. The rational person will choose policies that promise both freedom from pain and as long a life as possible; only if the man-in-the-street understands the theory and the operations of the policy will he, too, be able to see that it accomplishes both.

Conclusion: A Warning

This argument, that in an age-rationing system, direct termination of the lives of the elderly more nearly achieves justice than denying them treatment, may seem to be of *reductio ad absurdum* form, but it is not. In a society characterized by substantial scarcity of resources, this contemporary analogue of ancient practices is the only fair response. However, this view does not—*repeat, NOT*—entail that contemporary society should impose age-rationing or exterminate those among its elderly who are in poor health. For one thing, it is by no means clear that rationing, either by denial of treatment or direct termination, is better than providing full medical care for all the elderly who wish it, even at the expense of other social goods. Age rationing is a rationally defensible policy only if the alleged scarcity is real and cannot be relieved without introducing still greater injustices. But it may well be that the very scarcity assumption that gives rise to the issue of justice in health care in the first place is not accurate. Certainly, some of the pressure on resources could be reduced by pruning waste and by greater attention to patients' actual desire for care; a substantial amount of health care expense attributable to the paternalistic imposition of treatment and to "defensive medicine" practices by physicians seeking to protect themselves from legal liability could be avoided. More importantly, the degree of scarcity in health care resources is itself a function of larger distributive choices among various kinds of social goods, including education, art, defense, welfare, and so on; the position of contemporary society does not resemble the economically precarious position of most of the primitive societies in which direct-termination practices have developed. Consequently, the appropriate response to the apparent cost containment crisis in health care is not necessarily to devise just policies for enacting rationing, by age or in any other way, but to reconsider the societal priorities assigned various social goods. Given a world very much like the present one, it may be asked, what ceiling would parties to the original position assign to health care? This might obviate the necessity for rationing at all.

Second, a redistributive policy cannot be just without adequate guarantees that resources will, in fact, be redistributed as required. To deprive the elderly of health care without reassigning the savings in the form of health care for younger age groups is not just, and ought not to be advertised in this way. Inasmuch as the erratic age rationing practiced in the United States (perhaps unlike that in a closed system, such as the British National Health Service[44]) is not tied directly to redistribution of this care to others, it can hardly be described as just, but rather the product of ordinary, socially entrenched age bias. Furthermore, a just rationing system requires a background of just institutions to ensure its operation, and neither the United States nor Britain can boast a full set of these—nor, for that matter, can any of the primitive or historical societies mentioned at the outset. Consequently, although I believe there is a cogent argument for the moral preferability of age rationing that involves voluntary but socially encouraged killing or self-killing of the elderly as their infirmities overcome them, in preference to the medical abandonment they would otherwise face, this is in no way a recommendation for the introduction of such practices in our present world. As Daniels remarks, if the basic institutions of a given society do not comply with acceptable principles of distributive justice, then rationing by age may make things worse[45]—and surely age rationing by direct-termination practices could make things very much worse indeed. Thus, while I think direct-termination practices would be just in a scarcity-characterized ideal world, I also think we should cast a skeptical eye on the sorts of arbitrary, unthinking age rationing we are toying with now.

Notes

1. Euripides, *Suppliants* 1109, as quoted by [pseudo-]Plutarch in "A Letter of Condolence to Apollonius," 110C, in *Plutarch's Moralia*, tr. Frank Cole Babbitt (London: William Heinemann; Cambridge, Mass.: Harvard University Press, 1928), II, 153.

2. Colorado's Governor Richard D. Lamm was widely (mis)quoted in March 1984 as claiming that the elderly terminally ill "have a duty to die," engendering extremely vigorous controversy. Lamm's own account of what he actually did say appears in *The New Republic* for August 27, 1984, as well as in a variety of speech and press corrections about that time.

3. *Republic* III 406C.

4. Book II, "Their Care of the Sick and Euthanasia," tr. H. V. S. Ogden (Northbrook, Ill.: AHM, 1949), p. 57.

5. Friedrich Nietzsche, *The Twilight of the Idols.* In *The Complete Works of Friedrich Nietzsche,* edited by Oscar Levy, translated by Anthony M. Ludovici. London: George Allen & Unwin, 1927, p. 88.

6. See Alexander H. Leighton and Charles C. Hughes, "Notes on Eskimo Patterns of Suicide," *Southwestern Journal of Anthropology* 11 (1955) pp. 327–38, for a description of suicide practices from Yuit Eskimo informants on St. Lawrence Island, Alaska, and a survey of the literature on Eskimo suicide generally.

7. This practice is movingly depicted in the Imamura film *The Ballad of Narayama,* but there remains considerable controversy concerning whether the practice in fact has historical roots or is the product of legend imported at a later period.

8. The Hippocratic oath reflects the opposition of what was a minority school to this practice. See L. Edelstein, "The Hippocratic Oath: Text, Translation, and Interpretation," in *Supplements to the Bulletin of the History of Medicine* no. 1 (1943), and in *Ancient Medicine: Selected Papers of Ludwig Edelstein,* Oswei Temkin and C. Lillian Temkin, eds. (1967), both Baltimore, Md.: The Johns Hopkins Press. Also see Danielle Gourevitch, "Suicide Among the Sick in Classical Antiquity," *Bulletin of the History of Medicine* 43 (1969), pp. 501–18.

9. See Gitta Sereny, *Into That Darkness: From Mercy Killing to Mass Murder* (New York: McGraw-Hill 1974), for an account of the development of "euthanasia" policies under Hitler and their relationship to the mass extermination programs, and Robert Jay Lifton, *The Nazi Doctors: Medical Killing and the Psychology of Genocide* (New York: Basic Books, 1986).

10. S. Jay Olshansky and A. Brian Ault, "The Fourth Stage of the Epidemiologic Transition: The Age of Delayed Degenerative Diseases," this volume.

11. Norman Daniels, "Justice Between Age Groups: Am I My Parents' Keeper?," *Milbank Memorial Fund Quarterly* 61 (1983), p. 515.

12. U.S. Senate Special Committee on Aging, *Aging America, Trends and Projections,* 1984, p. 70.

13. B. B. Torrey, "The Visible Costs of the Invisible Aged: The Fiscal Implications of the Growth in the Very Old," paper presented to the American Association for the Advancement of Science, New York, 1984, p. 1.

14. *Ibid.,* p. 6.

15. J. H. Schultz, *The Economics of Aging* (Belmont, Calif.: Wadsworth 1985), p. 140.

16. *Ibid.,* p. 73.

17. J. W. Rowe, "Health Care of the Elderly," *New England Journal of Medicine* 312 (1985), p. 831.

18. Rowe, *op. cit.,* p. 828, citing Sidney Katz *et al.,* "Active Life Expectancy," *New England Journal of Medicine* 309 (Nov. 17, 1983): 1218–24.

19. James Lubitz and Ronald Prihoda, "The Use and Costs of Medicare Services in the Last Two Years of Life," *Health Care Financing Review* 5 (Spring 1984) 3, p. 119.

20. Anne A. Scitovsky, " 'The High Cost of Dying': What Do the Data Show?", *Milbank Memorial Fund Quarterly/Health and Society* 62 (1984): 591–608, p. 598, using data from Lubitz and Prihoda, *op. cit.,* Fig. 2, p. 124.

21. W. Hines, *Chicago Sun–Times,* Feb. 9, 1983, p. 72.

22. Daniels, *op. cit.,* passim.

23. John Rawls, *A Theory of Justice* (Cambridge, Mass.: Harvard University Press 1971), sec. 24, p. 138.

24. Parties to the original position are not only hypothetical but ahistorical, having no knowledge of what historical period they live in. The parties described here, however, seem to have an extraordinary amount of information about health care costs in the 1980s. But this is simply part of the general information such parties are assumed to have (see Rawls's *A Theory of Justice,* sec. 24, p. 142); it can be assumed that they also have similarly detailed information about health care costs in other historical periods, both before and after the 1980s. Regardless of the degree of technological development of medicine in these historical periods, however, in all periods providing extensive care in end-of-life illness is more costly than denying care or directly terminating life; hence, in all of these periods, the age-rationing problem will look very much like it does now.

25. See H. J. Aaron and W. B. Schwartz, *The Painful Prescription: Rationing Hospital Care* (Washington, D.C.: The Brookings Institution 1984) for an account of age-rationing in Britain.

26. I have in mind non-medically-indicated age ceilings for heart transplants at Stanford, waiting lists in the Veterans' Administration system for hip replacements, Medicaid's reduction of physical therapy for nursing home patients from twice daily to once daily, and the like.

27. Health care expenditures for the elderly are estimated to reach 3.3 percent of the GNP in 1984, or nearly one-third of the 10.5 percent of the GNP that represents all health care. See D. R. Waldo and H. C. Lazenby, "Demographic Characteristics and Health Care Use and Expenditures by the Aged in the United States: 1977–1984," *Health Care Financing Review* 6(1) (Fall 1984), p. 8.

28. Olshansky and Ault, *op. cit.*, pp. 4–5.

29. The "normal life span" is not to be confused with the "average life span," which 50 percent of the people do not reach and 50 percent exceed. The concept of "normal life span" employed by Daniels and others is not defined as a statistical notion, but appears to have to do with the rough boundary between middle and old age or between young old age and old old age.

30. See C. R. Fisher, "Differences by Age Groups in Health Care Spending," *Health Care Financing Review* 2(5) Spring 1980, p. 69, fig. 1.

31. John K. Iglehart, "The Cost of Keeping the Elderly Well," *National Journal* 10(43) (Oct. 28, 1978) p. 1729.

32. Rowe, *op. cit.*, p. 830.

33. See Waldo and Lazenby, *op. cit.*, p. 2.

34. James F. Fries, M.D., "Aging, Natural Death, and the Compression of Morbidity," *New England Journal of Medicine* Vol. 303, No. 3 (July 17, 1980), pp.130–35.

35. Edward L. Schneider and Jacob A. Brody, "Aging, Natural Death, and the Compression of Morbidity: Another View," *New England Journal of Medicine* Vol. 309, No. 14 (October 6, 1983), pp. 854–55.

36. Fries, *op. cit.*, p. 135.

37. Rawls, *Theory of Justice*, sec. 26, p. 155.

38. Rawls, *Theory of Justice*, sec. 25, p. 145.

39. See My "Manipulated Suicide," in *Suicide: The Philosophical Issues,* M. Pabst Battin and David J. Mayo, eds. (New York: St. Martin's Press 1980), pp. 172–73.

40. Barrington, "Apologia for Suicide," in Battin and Mayo, *op. cit.*, p. 97.

41. Battin and Mayo, *op. cit.*, pp. 172–73.

42. Daniels, *op. cit.*, p. 513.

43. Victor Fuchs, " 'Though Much is Taken': Reflections on Aging, Health, and Medical Care," *Milbank Memorial Fund Quarterly* 62 (1984), pp. 151–52.

44. See Daniels, "Why Saying No to Patients in the United States is So Hard: Cost Containment, Justice, and Provider Autonomy," *New England Journal of Medicine* 314(21) (May 22, 1986), pp. 1380–1383.

45. Daniels, "Justice Between Age Groups," *op. cit.*, p. 519.

Comments

Daniel Wikler

Although the movement to establish a right to die has largely succeeded, few people other than Governor Lamm have been willing to speak publicly about a duty to die. Margaret P. Battin, however, has been one of those people, and her *Ethical Issues in Suicide* contains one of the first substantial contemporary discussions of the concept. That thoughtful book challenged the reader to support the common belief that no one owes it to others to die, and shows that the easiest arguments are easily countered. In her new paper, Professor Battin presents a deep, sophisticated argument in favor of the contrary, radical view. Although she presents reasons in the end to ignore the argument, and thus to uphold conventional medical morality, it is the radical argument that deserves our attention.

Professor Battin argues that a just society, and a just health care system, under certain conditions that do not now obtain, would attempt to engineer a social consensus in favor of suicide on the part of older patients with disabling, uncomfortable, expensive-to-treat terminal or chronic diseases. Hers is the most exciting kind of argument: big ideas in unexpected combination aiming to undermine conventional wisdom. It is theoretically informed, and presented clearly and precisely. This exactitude makes it possible for a commentator to take careful aim. I will argue that Professor Battin's conclusion does not—thank goodness—follow from her premise. My objections do not at all show, however, that conventional wisdom can ignore the trenchant arguments and unsettling questions posed by Professor Battin here and elsewhere.

My first objection will be familiar to those acquainted with the secondary literature on Rawls's *A Theory of Justice*. Rawls's grand argument was expressly intended to provide a way of deciding on the *basic structure* of the just society. There are several particular reasons, which I will not state here, for doubting that the Rawlsian apparatus is suited to deciding upon more specific moral issues. There is a difference between the general idea of people deciding what rules they favor before knowing whether they will win or lose as a result, and the particular apparatus of Rawls's Original Position. The former ought not to be credited with the philosophical power of the latter, which stands or falls on the success of its specific supporting arguments. Professor Battin, of course, cannot develop a background theory of comparable elegance in the context of this paper, but there must be the promise of one, and we must take into account the likelihood that it could be made good.

Let us proceed, however, by accepting Professor Battin's particular contractarian or hypothetical approach. She argues from two main premises: 1) Justice requires a shift of health care resources from the old to the young (taken over from Norman Daniels's analysis). 2) We are better off if our death is not preceded by long, painful, and debilitating illness.

Do these imply that justice requires us to encourage voluntary euthanasia at the time of approaching terminal illness? I think not. My response has five steps:

1. We must ask: How draconian must the shift of resources from old to young be? *Very*, according to Professor Battin, including even the means of palliation. Otherwise, she holds, we would not save enough to do very much for the young.

2. What is the remainder? This is the means of subsistence. Call it "bread and water." Professor Battin does not insist that this (or its monetary equivalent) must also be shifted to the young. Furthermore, Professor Battin says that merely denying treatment to the sick old does not do them in; they linger on.

It follows from this, and Professor Battin's other premises, that justice does not require the shift of bread and water. Therefore, it is consistent with justice that the sick old be permitted to live on, so long as they are given only the means of subsistence.

3. Why, then, would justice require us to engineer a social climate in which suicide at the onset of terminal illness is seen as a duty?

The answer cannot be that suicide would be *prudent* under those circumstances. For one thing, it might not be. Professor Battin argues that death not preceded by illness is better than death that follows a long illness, but this is quite different from the claim that death is better than illness. It all depends on the schedule. If I am to die on a certain date, let me be disease-free until then; but if I can live on diseased, it will often be in my interests to do so.

In any case, the Rawlsian apparatus generates principles for distributing goods between people. Deciding whether suicide is in one's own best interest is not a distributional question. People in the Original Position might individually agree (just because it is plausible) that suicide would be prudent and rational under certain conditions, but their concurrence would not lend support to the view that suicide would be required or encouraged in a just society.

Thus, we are left with the two premises, but not with the conclusion.

4. We should be clear on the difference between what might be called the "time to die" idea and Professor Battin's "duty to die."

The "time to die" claim, which I mean to represent Governor Lamm's position, is that the old should sometime decline to make use of health care resources *which are offered to them*. They will do this because they recognize that the resources could do much more good if used for others.

Professor Battin's first premise, however, denies these resources to the old and sick. It says that to offer the resources to them would be unjust. They would not have the opportunity to be self-denying. To be sure, the suicide decision would be voluntary (although encouraged) under Professor Battin's regime. But the only decision open to them is whether to kill themselves, *given that they have been denied curative or even palliative care*. My question, in any case, is why justice requires that this be encouraged.

5. Finally, we must distinguish between the society that prohibits or inhibits prudent, rational suicide, and the society that denies curative and palliative care and requires or encourages suicide over subsistence. The former may be undesirable for various reasons, but that is not what Professor Battin's argument seeks to demonstrate. Her conclusion is the latter.

Governor Lamm's controversial and stimulating remarks have been seen as a response to the "graying of America" and its concomitant increase in health care costs. This phenomenon, however, plays only a small role in Professor Battin's argument. I think that her approach applies with equal force to any terminal patient or chronic sufferer. It addresses issues that have been with us since the time that medicine became capable of keeping people alive, and continues her long-standing and important study of these problems.

As John Myles has recently shown, however, even the aging of the United States population presents us with no issues in medical ethics that are really new. Despite current fears and assumptions, there are not going to be newer, heavier burdens on people in their "productive" years. There will be more aged, but relatively fewer children. The burden of caring for the aged is simply and incompletely replacing the decreasing burden of caring for the young.

Why, then, does it suddenly seem appropriate to be talking about killing sick, old people? This, I think, is a political question, and deserves a political answer.

5

Medical Decision-Making, Dying, and Quality of Life Among the Elderly

John Collette
Peter Y. Windt

Introduction

THERE IS WIDESPREAD AGREEMENT that decisions about medical care for elderly patients should be concerned with the patient's quality of life, both at the level of individual patient care, and at the level of policy (Neu 1980). But, there is substantial disagreement about how quality of life should be evaluated and, once evaluated, how it should be weighed against potentially competing considerations, such as the value of prolonging life, or the need to ration limited medical resources. Nor is it clear how potential gains in some aspects of a patient's life are to be weighed against potential losses in other aspects, particularly when family, rather than individual needs and resources, are considered (Maddox 1975). Decisions to prolong the lives of the elderly typically view prolongation as the goal to be achieved without questioning whether the prolonged life is of satisfactory quality. Lissitz (1975), for example, says that the traditional goal of organizations that serve the elderly "is the prolongation through consistent medical, paramedical and social services of an effective life." Effective life need not be of satisfactory quality, of course.

The ideal approach to medical decision-making for the elderly patient involves clarification and substantial resolution of these normative issues. In the research described here, we begin the needed clarification and resolution by addressing the question: How do the participants in medical decisions about elderly patients view the importance of quality of life in making these decisions? Our aim is to understand more clearly the dynamics of the medical decision-making process, and the role that the decision-maker's assessments of quality of life play in the process. We intend this research to provide a background of information that will illuminate subsequent investigation of the normative issues identified above.

Following Neu's (1980:273) suggestion that basic information is needed regarding patients' preferences among various health outcomes, we have set the following objectives for the research reported here:

1. to determine, for a selected set of conditions, the impact of those conditions in quality of life as perceived by those who participate in medical decision-making for elderly patients;
2. to discover whether some groups of decision-makers tend to assess the prospective quality of life differently than do other groups;
3. to determine the importance of assessments of life quality in deciding whether to prolong life for elderly patients.

It should be emphasized here that, in this research, we take no stand on the merits or faults of various proposed analyses of quality of life, or of proposed indicators of quality of life. Our concern is not with the actual quality of life achieved by the elderly patient after a medical decision has been made and carried out, but with the role played by the decider's perception, while the decision is being made, of what that quality of life will be.

We employ some of the standard devices used to measure quality of life, including both tests for so-called *objective* quality of life (roughly speaking, those that measure the extent of approximation to normal health and function), and for *subjective* quality of life (those that measure psychological morale and life satisfaction). Our use of these indicators is to determine whether the life quality of the decision-maker, as measured against these standards, emerges as a reliable predictor of the way in which the decision-maker perceives prospective quality of life, and how that perception figures in arriving at a medical decision. The potential for confusion here is greatest where the decision-maker under investigation is, in fact, the elderly person about whom the decision is being made. In such cases, it is important not to confuse our appraisal of the life satisfaction of that elderly person with the person's own appraisal of his or her present quality of life, or of the perceived impact on his or her quality of life that would result from a decision about the course of care to be taken.

Those who take part in decisions about the health care of elderly patients can be divided (although not without remainder) into three major groups. First there are the elderly themselves, who participate in decisions about their own care, or the care of their spouses. Second, there are the young to middle-aged adults who participate in decisions about care for an elderly parent or parents-in-law. Finally, there are the health care providers who have elderly patients or clients.

In this analysis, we have selected populations from each of these three groups and have conducted interviews to obtain data from those respondents, specifically their responses to a set of questions about five conditions often experienced by elderly patients that we assume to adversely affect the quality of life of many of those patients. Within each group we wished to discover (a) whether there is variation or uniformity in the perceived impact on quality of life of each of the five conditions; (b) among those who agree in these perceptions, whether there is further agreement or variation in their willingness to accept that impact on their own lives in exchange for modest prolongation of life; (c) whether there is variation between willingness to accept each condition for oneself, and willingness to impose it on others for whom one might have decision-making responsibility; and finally, (d) the extent to which willingness to submit oneself or others to each condition is a function of the decider's current subjective life quality or perceived impacts of that condition on the quality of life.

Method of Study

Data for this research were collected during the summer of 1985. Telephone interviews were conducted with three groups of respondents: the elderly (those over 60), adults aged 35–55 with living elderly parents, and physicians with elderly patients. Respondents were selected through a computer-assisted random dialing procedure. Our initial sampling frame called for 200 elderly respondents, 100 middle-aged adults, and 50 physicians. The elderly and middle-aged samples were drawn separately from the general population of households in Utah with telephones. The sample of physicians was drawn from the population of licensed general practitioners. Interviews were completed with 199 elderly respondents, 107 middle-aged adults with living, elderly parents, and 49 physicians with elderly patients.

Respondents in each of the three samples were questioned about general potential health care decisions and their likely effect on life quality as well as background characteristics, current health and life quality, living conditions, and the like.

Of particular concern for this analysis were the ways in which the three samples perceived the likely effect on life quality of medical decisions that the elderly and their families might face at some time in the future. Variables related to potential life quality examined in this analysis include:

1. For the elderly sample:
   a. current subjective life quality, or morale, measured by the Philadelphia Geriatric Center (PGC) Morale Scale (Lawton 1972, 1975);
   b. the perceived threat to their life quality of five healthy outcomes associated with the elderly: bed confinement, dependency on a respirator or other life support mechanism, constant pain, incontinence, living in a nursing home;
   c. willingness to undergo each of these health decision outcomes in order to extend life for a year;
   d. willingness to have a loved one (e.g., spouse, sibling) undergo each health outcome in order to extend his or her life for a year.
2. For the middle-aged sample:
   a. current subjective life quality (PGC Scale);
   b. perceived threat to their own life quality of each of the five health outcomes;
   c. willingness to undergo each of the five outcomes in order to extend life for a year;
   d. willingness to have a loved one (e.g., parent) undergo each outcome in order to extend his or her life for a year.
3. For the sample of physicians:
   a. current subjective life quality (PGC Scale);
   b. perceived threat to their own life quality of each of the five health outcomes;
   c. perceived threat to the life quality of the average elderly patient of the five outcomes;
   d. willingness to undergo each outcome in order to extend life for a year;
   e. willingness to have a loved one undergo each outcome in order to extend his or her life for a year;
   f. willingness to have an elderly patient undergo each outcome in order to extend his or her life for a year.

Although the PGC scale was developed for use with elderly populations, we also used it with our middle-aged and physician samples for purposes of comparability.

Findings

Perceived Threat

In Table 5.1, we show data regarding respondents' perceptions of the impact of decision outcomes on life quality. Respondents in each of the three samples were asked how each outcome would affect their life quality. Possible responses included "much worse," "worse," "about the same," and, if volunteered, "better." Not surprisingly, most respondents felt that life quality would be worsened by the decision outcomes. Table 5.1 shows the percentage of each of the samples who reported that their life quality would be made "much worse" by each of the decision outcomes. Respirator or other life support dependency and bed confinement were seen as the outcomes most threatening to life quality. Somewhat lower proportions of each sample viewed pain, incontinence, and nursing home residence as making their life quality much worse than at present.

For the elderly sample, both men and women viewed respirator dependency as most threatening to life quality, with over eighty percent of each sex perceiving respirator dependency as making life quality much worse. Constant pain was perceived as the least threatening outcome for both elderly women and men.

For four of the five outcomes, slightly higher proportions of elderly men than of women perceived life quality as much worse; only with regard to respirator dependency did a higher proportion of women than men perceive life quality as much worse. Elderly men and women also showed considerable agreement about each outcome. The percentages reported in Table 5.1 for the elderly sample are quite similar for men and women, with an average gender difference of less than four percent for the five outcomes. Also, the average number of outcomes perceived as making life quality much worse were very similar for both sexes in the elderly sample (3.31 and 3.59, see last column).

Among the middle-aged respondents, the five outcomes posed somewhat less threat to life quality than they did for the elderly sample. Middle-aged men were less likely than their elderly counterparts to perceive each of the outcomes as making their life quality much worse. Middle-aged men perceived respirator dependency as fairly threatening to life quality, but only about half perceived life quality as being much worse under conditions of bed confinement (56.4 percent), constant pain (53.8 percent) or nursing home residence (54.5 percent). Just over one-third (36.4 percent) perceived incontinence as a major threat compared to two-thirds of elderly men.

Middle-aged women, except regarding respirator dependency, saw

Table 5.1 Percent Perceiving Each Decision Outcome as Making Life Quality "Much Worse," and Mean Number of Outcomes Perceived as Being "Much Worse," by Sample and Gender

Sample and Gender	Decision Outcome					Number of Outcomes Perceived "Much Worse" $(\overline{X})$
	Bedridden %	On a Respirator %	In Constant Pain %	Incontinent %	In a Nursing Home %	
Elderly						
Men (N = 78)	76.1	83.3	61.0	67.8	67.5	3.31
Women (N = 121)	69.4	84.6	55.2	63.0	67.3	3.59
Middle-aged						
Men (N = 51)	56.4	74.3	53.8	36.4	54.5	2.72
Women (N = 56)	68.8	70.6	68.8	43.1	62.6	3.13
Physicians (N = 49)						
For self	83.0	90.6	44.9	53.1	54.2	3.23
For average elderly patient	61.2	85.4	53.1	43.8	23.3	2.66

each decision outcome more similarly to the elderly. Middle-aged men responded "much worse" to an average of 2.72 out of five outcomes while women in this age group averaged 3.13 outcomes out of five perceived as making life quality much worse.

Physicians showed a similar pattern to the elderly when judging the impact of each outcome on their own life quality. Relatively high proportions of the physicians saw respirator dependency and bed confinement as making their life quality much worse. Just over half saw incontinence (53.1 percent) and nursing home residence (54.2 percent) as having that degree of threat to their life quality. Just under half (44.9 percent) perceived constant pain as a major threat to life quality.

Physicians perceived respirator dependency to be nearly as threatening to the life quality of the elderly as to their own life quality, and constant pain was seen as more threatening to the elderly (53.1 percent) than to themselves. Fewer physicians saw bed confinement as a major threat to life quality for the elderly (61.2 percent) than as a major threat to their own life quality (83.0 percent). Incontinence was also perceived as less of a threat to the elderly. Regarding nursing home residence, more than twice as many physicians saw a major threat to their own life quality (54.2 percent) than as a major threat to the life quality of the elderly (23.3 percent).

Willingness to Undergo Outcomes

Although the data presented in Table 5.1 indicate that the five health outcomes pose considerable threat to life quality, respondents from all three samples showed some degree of willingness to accept each of those outcomes if it would extend their lives for a year or more. Respondents were also asked if they would decide to have a loved one undergo each outcome if it would extend the life of the loved one. In addition to these questions, physicians were asked for the same decision regarding an elderly patient. Table 5.2 shows the responses of each subsample for these questions.

Data in Table 5.2 show a pattern reflective of that in Table 5.1, that is, the greater the perceived threat to life quality a decision outcome represents, the less likely were respondents to desire life extension at the cost of that outcome whether for self or for others. For example, respirator dependency and bed confinement were viewed as relatively threatening to life quality. Table 5.2 shows that relatively few respondents would undergo these outcomes to extend their own lives for a year. Relatively higher proportions of each group would accept pain, incontinence, and nursing home residence.

In general, each age-gender group was more willing to accept each

Table 5.2 Percent Who Would Extend Life at the Cost of Each Decision Outcome for Self and Loved Ones, and Mean Number of Outcomes Agreed to by Sample and Gender

Sample and Gender	Bedridden %	On a Respirator %	In Constant Pain %	Incontinent %	In a Nursing Home %	Number of Outcomes Agreed to ($\overline{X}$)
Elderly Men						
For self	19.0	22.7	37.3	39.1	50.7	1.56
For loved one	39.6	30.3	41.8	45.4	62.6	1.86
Elderly Women						
For self	18.8	10.0	36.2	47.6	51.0	1.41
For loved one	48.0	25.0	40.5	56.0	64.5	1.74
Middle-aged Men						
For self	9.5	18.8	50.5	62.1	47.3	1.80
For loved one	18.9	25.0	33.0	64.2	52.7	1.81
Middle-aged Women						
For self	17.5	19.0	55.4	62.1	43.4	1.90
For loved one	35.0	30.5	29.7	64.1	63.6	2.10
Physicians						
For self	30.6	16.2	47.5	65.9	61.4	2.02
For loved one	32.5	18.9	35.0	70.7	72.7	2.06
For elderly patient	36.1	19.4	35.0	65.9	72.7	2.12

of the outcomes for a loved one than for themselves. The last column of Table 5.2 shows the average number of outcomes agreed to for self and loved ones and, for the physician sample, for an elderly patient. Elderly men and women in particular show a discrepancy between what they would accept for self and for a loved one. Middle-aged women also agree to more of the outcomes for a loved one (1.90 vs. 2.10 in Table 5.2, last column). Middle-aged men showed nearly identical levels of average acceptance for self and loved ones. Physicians also showed a great deal of similarity between their average acceptance for self, for a loved one, and for an elderly patient.

Comparing the average numbers of outcomes to which respondents agreed also shows some interesting differences across samples. The elderly were least accepting, overall, of the medical outcomes. The middle-aged were somewhat more accepting, and the physicians even more so.

Decisions for the Elderly

The configuration of perceptions and decisions regarding life extension that concern us most in the analysis is that configuration regarding the (potential) elderly patient. This involves: for the elderly, their self-perceptions of current life quality, life quality threat, and willingness to undergo each outcome; for the middle-aged their perceived life quality, life quality threat, and life extension decision for a loved one; for the physicians, their perceived life quality, life quality threat and life extension decision for an elderly patient. Tables 5.3-5.5 report the cross-tabulations of the pertinent variables for each subsample.

Table 5.3 shows the cross-tabulation of life extension decision for each outcome with current life quality and perceived threat to life quality of each outcome. Except for incontinence, there was a curvilinear relationship between current life quality and willingness to undergo each outcome, with those in good morale and in low morale being less willing to accept outcomes. Those with moderate morale were more accepting of each outcome. Regarding threat to life quality, there was a clear negative pattern with higher threat associated with lower acceptance.

Table 5.4 shows the same cross-tabulations for the middle-aged sample. Here, each of the decision outcomes shows a clearly positive relationship between current life quality and willingness to have a loved one undergo the outcome. The better the middle-aged respondent's morale, the greater his or her willingness to accept the decision outcome for a loved one. Perceived threat of each outcome, as in the elderly sample, was negative in its influence on outcome decisions; the greater the perceived threat to life quality, the less the likelihood of willingness to have a loved one undergo the decision outcome.

Table 5.3   Percent of Elderly Sample Willing to Undergo Each Decision Outcome by
Current Life Quality, and Perceived Threat to Life Quality of Each Outcome

Current Life Quality and Threat to Life Quality	Percent Willing to Undergo Being:				
	Bedridden	On a Respirator	In Constant Pain	Incontinent	In A Nursing Home
Current Life Quality					
High	11.4	12.8	35.1	24.3	43.2
Moderate	18.8	14.3	40.9	41.8	51.5
Low	16.4	12.7	38.7	43.5	41.0
	Q = −.24	Q = −.02	Q = −.09	Q = −.40	Q = −.05
Threat to Life Quality					
High	13.2	7.7	36.0	27.4	33.7
Low	23.5	34.6	50.7	58.6	74.5
	Q = −.35	Q = −.72	Q = −.41	Q = −.58	Q = −.70

Q = correlation coefficient

Table 5.5 shows similar cross-tabulation for the sample of physicians. Here a clear pattern can be seen. Both current life quality and the perceived threat to life quality, whether the physician's own, or his or her elderly patient's, were negatively associated with each decision outcome. There was also a great deal of similarity between the physician's decisions regarding a loved one and those regarding an elderly patient.

Discussion and Conclusions

The findings presented above indicate a number of respects in which the outcome of medical decisions about care for elderly patients may not be responsive to the preferences of those patients. Willingness to extend life at the cost of imposing one of the outcomes studied is, to some extent, a function of one's perception of the degree of threat to life quality represented by that outcome. Since physicians, the middle-aged, and even the spouses of elderly patients often will perceive that degree of threat differently than the elderly patient, there is a risk that some of the medical decisions in which members of these groups have strong influence will not conform to the patient's wishes. Further, since willingness to extend life at the cost of imposing these outcomes is a function of the morale (subjective life quality) of the

Table 5.4　Percent of Middle-Aged Sample Willing to Have a Parent Undergo Each
Decision Outcome by Current Life Quality, and Perceived Threat to Life
Quality of Each Outcome

Current Life Quality and Threat to Life Quality	Percent Willing to Have Parent Undergo Being:				
	Bedridden	On a Respirator	In Constant Pain	Incontinent	In A Nursing Home
Life Quality					
High	41.0	35.1	37.0	74.1	64.7
Low	21.2	18.2	23.3	46.7	56.2
	Q = .28	Q = .42	Q = .32	Q = .53	Q = .18
Threat to Life Quality					
High	18.3	20.3	27.5	58.2	46.9
Low	41.0	50.0	36.8	69.4	73.2
	Q = −.50	Q = −.59	Q = −.20	Q = −.18	Q = −.46

Q = correlation coefficient

decider, we may expect discrepancies in willingness to prolong life
where the morale of the elderly patient is substantially better or worse
than the morale of health care providers or significant others participating in the decision.

Also indicated in our finding is a fairly widespread tendency to be
willing to impose conditions on others that one would not be willing
to accept for oneself. An interesting exception to this tendency is the
case of pain, where respondents were generally more reluctant to
impose the condition on others (even though they tended to perceive
it as *least* threatening to life quality) than to accept it for themselves.
For four of the outcomes studied, then, even where the elderly
patient and others participating in medical decisions agree about the
threat to life quality and are similar in terms of morale, there will be
some tendency for the others to advocate an outcome that the patient
is unwilling to accept. In the case of pain, there will be some tendency
to withhold an outcome that the patient would be willing to accept.

Overall, the data suggest that where the result of a medical decision
is not compatible with the elderly patient's wishes, there is a greater
likelihood that outcomes will be imposed on the patient that the
patient does not regard as acceptable, than that life will not be
prolonged in order to avoid outcomes that the patient might regard as
acceptable. In light of the fact that cost of care for elderly patients is by
far highest during the last year of life, these findings offer some

Table 5.5 Percent of Physicians Willing to Have An Elderly Patient Undergo Each Decision Outcome by Physician's Current Life Quality, Perceived Threat to Physician's Life Quality of Each Outcome, and Perceived Threat to Elderly Patient's Life Quality of Each Outcome

Current Life Quality and Threat to Life Quality	Percent Willing to Have Elderly Patient Undergo Being:				
	Bedridden	On a Respirator	In Constant Pain	Incontinent	In A Nursing Home
Current Life Quality					
High	31.3	13.0	31.8	73.1	84.6
Low	68.1	31.3	41.2	55.6	88.2
	Q = −.28	Q = −.50	Q = −.20	Q = −.37	Q = −.15
Threat to Own Life Quality					
High	34.5	17.1	15.8	36.4	83.3
Low	40.0	50.0	55.0	95.5	88.9
	Q = −.21	Q = −.66	Q = −.73	Q = −.95	Q = −.17
Threat to Life Quality of Elderly					
High	34.8	12.5	27.3	31.6	77.8
Low	33.3	66.7	47.1	91.7	86.2
	Q = −.03	Q = −.87	Q = −.41	Q = −.92	Q = −.12

Q = correlation coefficient

support for the view that lower health care costs might result from making medical decisions that conform more closely to the preferences of the elderly patients themselves.

But, of course, these results do not answer any normative questions about the role that considerations of quality of life should play in medical decision-making for elderly patients. If one places primary ethical emphasis on the importance of the patient's right to accept or reject medical care (a model emphasizing informed voluntary consent), then the findings above may indicate factors that could lead others involved in medical decisions to violate that right of the elderly patient—that is, health care providers and family might be seen as illegitimately tending to impose life-prolonging care, which the patients themselves would prefer to forego. On the other hand, it could be argued that elderly patients tend to be too fearful, and misappraise the impact on life quality of the conditions studied. In that case, if one emphasizes the ethical importance of prolonging life of acceptable quality for as long as possible, it will seem appropriate for family and health care providers to impose some of these conditions against the (unrealistically founded) wishes of the elderly patient. And there are still other possibilities. For example, it could be argued that *regardless of impact on quality of life*, family members have a duty to preserve the lives of their loved ones, and physicians a duty to preserve life. Our findings indicate, however, that to the extent that appraisals of quality of life do have an ethically significant role to play in medical decision-making for elderly patients, it is likely that a number of these decisions are ethically flawed.

Much remains to be done in subsequent studies. In addition to enlarging data already gathered by studying a larger and more varied population, the following questions need to be addressed:

1. What other outcomes of medical care are perceived to be significant to quality of life, and how much agreement or disagreement is there among potential decision-makers about the impact of these outcomes on life quality? It seems clear, for example, that loss of one or more senses, loss of cognitive function, loss of independence, loss of social relationships, as well as other negative outcomes should be studied along with the five considered in this pilot study.

2. What other groups are involved in health care for elderly patients, and what is the character of their perceptions of quality of life, and willingness to impose or withhold outcomes of care for elderly patients? Nurses who care for elderly patients should be included in further studies, and it might be useful to consider the attitudes of administrators of health care institutions (both short-term and long-term) and of resource allocation agencies such as insurance companies.

3. Whose perceptions of impact on life quality are accurate? It could be argued that the elderly tend to be too fearful, or alternatively, that the middle-aged tend to be insensitive to the impact of some conditions on quality of life. As one step toward resolving these questions, a longitudinal study could show whether prospective, retrospective, and contemporaneous appraisals of the impact of an outcome on life quality agree or disagree.

4. What explanation is there for the discrepancy between willingness to accept an outcome for oneself and willingness to impose it on another?

5. How well do actual medical decisions and their dynamics conform to the models established by hypothetical deliberations of the sort involved in this study?

6. What role, if any, is played in evaluation of life quality and in decision-making by the need to eliminate cognitive dissonance?

Data pertinent to all these questions are needed if we are to understand the dynamics of medical decision-making well enough to decide whether it is typically responsive to the elderly patient's needs (which may or may not be identical with the patient's preferences), or whether it tends to impose overtreatment or undertreatment.

References

Lawton, M. P. 1972. "The Dimensions of Morale." In *Research Planning and Action for the Elderly*. D. Kent et al. New York: Behavioral Publications.
———. 1975. "The Philadelphia Center Morale Scale." *Journal of Gerontology* 30:85–89.
Lissitz, S. 1970. "Theoretical Conceptions of Institutional and Community Care." *Gerontologist* 12:220–24.
Maddox, G. L. 1975. "Families as Context and Resource in Chronic Illness." In *Long Term Care*, S. Sherwood, New York: Spectrum Publications.
Neu, C. R. 1980. "Individual Preferences for Life and Health: Misuses and Possible Uses." In *Values and Long-Term Care*, R. A. Kane and R. L. Kane. eds. Lexington, Mass.: D.C. Heath.

Comments

Dennis W. Jahnigen

THERE IS GROWING CONCERN about the manner in which medical care decisions for the elderly are made. One reason is the perception that care strategies providing minimal or no actual benefit to the elderly are often utilized. Another concern is the sense that medical therapies are frequently employed that are in opposition to the wishes of the elderly patient, particularly with regard to advanced life support technologies. Finally, and by no means the least potent force prompting concern, is a sense that the resources currently expended on health care for the elderly perhaps ought not to be spent.

There would appear to be several principles on which most of us would agree in making medical care decisions both with and for the elderly individual. In general, we would opt for strategies that preserve survival. This is not without modification, however, as few would not include some measures of "quality of life" in their consideration. Valid or not, there is widespread assumption that the "quality of life" of the elderly person is not as good as the "quality of life" of younger individuals. Another principle we would support in general is the respect for individual values, preferences, and choices. This is consonant with the widely accepted principle in contemporary American society that the patient has the prerogative to accept or decline any type of recommended medical care including life-sustaining treatments. Modifications to this principle become significant when the patient has diminished capacity to understand the implications of treatment and nontreatment.

As the elderly grow in numbers, and the technological capabilities of medical care increase, it becomes increasingly important to better understand how medical decisions are made and the degree to which the above principles are employed. It is in this context that the current study of Drs. Collette and Windt is most relevant.

Few investigators have chosen to explore the complex process whereby medical care decisions are formulated. What we have learned about such decisions provides some cause for concern. The studies, in general, support the role of "quality of life" as a determinant in physician recommendations for diagnostic and therapeutic interventions. How and by whom this "quality" is measured appears to be highly variable. In a study by Pearlman, et al.,[1] the authors found a variable perception of the patient's quality of life by the physicians presented with a hypothetical elderly patient with respiratory failure. Thirty percent of the physicians opting for intubation utilized the man's quality of life as the reason to place the patient on a ventilator, while half of the physicians who would not intubate the patient used that same quality of life principle to justify withholding ventilatory support. A study by Wolff, et al.,[2] regarding opinions of physicians and nurses regarding the appropriate level of care for patients in a university affiliated nursing home, demonstrated significant discordance, with the nurses favoring much less aggressive intervention for patients in real clinical situations. Bedell and Delbanco[3] interviewed survivors of cardiopulmonary resuscitation and found a very low correlation between the physician's opinion about a patient's desire for resuscitation, and the preference actually expressed by the patient. Of patients who were resuscitated, only nineteen percent had previously discussed this possibility with their physician. However, Snow and Atwood[4] have shown that 84 percent of elderly patients living in a retirement community had very definite opinions on the care that they would choose if death was imminent. There was significant heterogeneity expressed. While 56 percent wanted only comfort care should death be imminent, seven percent chose all available measures including cardiopulmonary resuscitation to give every chance for survival.

Drs. Collette and Windt in their preliminary studies have asked the questions, "What is the importance of assessment of quality of life in deciding whether to prolong life for elderly patients?" and "What role does the morale of the person making the quality of life assessment play in influencing the likelihood they will advocate a specific type of therapeutic intervention?" They conducted telephone interviews on hypothetical negative changes in health status with a group of elderly people living at home, middle-aged individuals with elderly parents, and physicians who care for elderly patients. Respondents were questioned as to how they viewed a negative change in health status for themselves, for a loved one, and for an elderly person, and comparisons were made within and among these groups.

It is important to be aware of the potential sources of misinformation in such a study before we can safely interpret its results. The average ages of the elderly individuals and their current health status were not reported. One would also like to know what prior experience respondents had with certain of these interventions such as respirators or nursing home care. It is likely that few persons have experience with such interventions and have false assumptions about the actual utility of such therapies. For example, nationally, one-third of all patients admitted to nursing homes subsequently improve enough to return to their own homes. In some institutions, this is as high as 50 percent. Most laymen estimate that only a small percentage of people ever return home from nursing homes. With incontinence, likewise, factual information about what it represents would significantly influence its acceptability in any given circumstance. Incontinence can be episodic or continuous. With specific therapies, it can be mitigated, and often with appropriate clothing and collecting devices, an individual is able to function in a normal fashion without embarrassment or limitation on their activity. The elderly respondent may have known of one or perhaps of no acquaintances who were ever on a ventilator and, thus, have attitudes based on misinformation. The physician respondent group, on the other hand, may have hundreds of experiences with each of the health status changes. For them, this should allow for a more realistic assessment of the likely impact on any specific individual's observed quality of life and, at the same time, make it more difficult to generalize for the "average" elderly person.

Another problem that mandates cautious interpretation of the results of the paper is that of sampling bias. The elderly respondents were, by their very participation in the study, mentally intact with moderately good health status as they were at home and willing to participate in a long telephone survey. They were not necessarily experiencing or facing major changes in health status. One would like to know how many patients declined to participate and for what reasons. In addition, the strength of comparing what the physician respondent group would advocate for a "typical" elderly patient, with the responses of a healthy community dwelling population is limited. This was not a cohort of physicians caring for this respondent cohort of elderly individuals.

A third factor mitigating the analysis of the study data is that respondent groups were provided a hypothetical health status change for consideration. There may very well be a significant difference between actual and stated behavior. The elderly, in fact, were asked to comment on decisions that it is unlikely they would ever be in a position to make. Only five percent of people above the age of 65 are in long-term care or acute care institutions at any one time. Although 20 percent of people above the age of 85 are in nursing homes, the vast majority remain in their homes, or are briefly hospitalized prior to death. The more remote the event is from an actual situation, the less likely the respondents' view is to be consistent with their behavior at such time as a choice is required. Finally, and perhaps most importantly, it is hazardous to move from measurement of normative values expressed in a hypothetical situation to inferences regarding individual decisions in a true clinical setting. Such results may be illustrative, intriguing, and provocative, but must be interpreted cautiously.

Even with these caveats, however, these data reveal interesting points. First, the elderly seem to fear dependency health status changes to a greater degree than the middle-aged or physician cohorts. Physicians agree with the elderly cohort that being bedridden, on a ventilator, or in constant pain are major negative health outcomes. Physicians, however, judged incontinence or residence in a nursing home to be much less negative for the elderly patient than the elderly group did itself. This may well reflect differences of experience with elderly who actually had the disability.

Another interesting observation is that both the elderly cohort and middle-aged cohort generally were much more willing to have a loved one undergo a negative intervention than they were for themselves. For physicians, there was remarkable consistency in what they would be willing to accept for themselves, for a loved one or for an elderly patient. This can be interpreted to support the position that physicians are likely to recommend the same care for elderly persons that they would accept for themselves or a loved one. Another very interesting finding of Collette and Windt is that, among all groups, the morale of the respondent was related to the conditions they hypothetically would accept for an elderly patient. For some conditions, the better the morale of the respondent group, the less acceptable a negative health status was. This suggests that the more real the necessity of one of the interventions to survive, the more acceptable it appears.

In their summary, the authors make a number of suggestions for future work. One of the most important is the degree to which actual medical decisions conform to the hypothetical models that the authors studied. This is an extremely important point, because group average attitudes about hypothetical situations may be substantially different than behavior in specific clinical situations.

Concomitant with studies such as Collette and Windt advocate is the need for change in the educational process for future physicians in geriatric medical care decision-making. At many medical schools and residency training programs, the traditional algorithm for medical decision-making is being modified to better suit the heterogeneity of the values of the elderly population. This process advocates a very individualized assessment of both the patient's value system, quality of life judged by the patient *him or herself,* and the physician's judgment as to the relative efficacy of any therapeutic intervention for a specific patient. This type of process may offer the best opportunity to avoid the "imposition" of care on people who do not desire it. It is a process that can be undertaken in a number of specific circumstances. These include: caring for an elderly patient who is facing an imminent decline in health status, presence of terminal disease, entry into a nursing home, presence of multiple chronic debilitating diseases, or even the presence of extreme old age itself where there is increasing likelihood of catastrophic event.

This process includes the following steps:

1. *Value Inventory.* A value inventory is information acquired in the context of a primary care relationship between a physician and an elderly patient. The patient offers, or the physician inquires as to the patient's own value system. This includes a sense of where the patient sees him or herself in the course of his own existence. Does he see himself coming to the end of his life? The ways in which the patient answers this and similar questions will help describe, in a broad way, his own personal value system. Information about the circumstances under which a patient might not want to live can be obtained at this time. Without this information, a physician and family members are left with only their own suppositions about what the patient might want in an emergency situation. The difference in views by these groups toward certain health status changes demonstrated by Collette and Windt point out the importance of obtaining this information in advance from the person most directly affected.

2. *Patient Expectations From the Medical Encounter.* Patients come into a medical relationship with differing expectations. While some genuinely want a cure, others simply want relief of symptoms, an explanation, sympathy, or validation of their worth as a human being by virtue of occupying a physician's attention. When a conscious effort is not made to discern the patient's expectations, there is a good possibility of misunderstanding by the physician.

3. *Establish the Medical Facts.* In this step, the factual medical issues are determined. What is the diagnosis, the natural history, the therapies available, and the physician's determination of the relative value of any of these options for this particular patient?
4. *Reconciliation.* This very important part of the process allows for negotiation between the patient and doctor about what is possible, desirable, permissible by the patient, and ultimately leads to an agreed upon mutually acceptable outcome. The patient may advocate an outcome that the physician is ethically unable to provide. The physician may advocate an intervention that is unacceptable to the patient. This resolution of any disagreements is critical to a satisfactory medical relationship.
5. *Strategy Development.* Finally, a plan is evolved. This can be diagnostic, life-sustaining, palliative, rehabilitative, experimental, or some similar type of strategy. Each strategy has different measures of success so that "failing to cure" a terminal patient would not necessarily be considered an unsatisfactory medical encounter if the patient's autonomy and dignity were preserved.

This type of systematic approach to the medical encounter arguably provides the best possible way of both allowing the patient to define the quality of his own existence and the acceptability of various outcomes, and of the medical professional to faithfully discharge his responsibility to offer the most effective medical attention possible.

One hopes that the work of Drs. Collette and Windt and similar studies will help clarify the degree to which this idealized paradigm of the medical encounter actually occurs.

Notes

1. Pearlman, R. A., T. S. Inui, and W. B. Carter. "Variability in Physician Bioethical Decision Making." *Annals of Internal Medicine* 97:420 (1982).

2. Wolff, M. L., S. Smolen, and L. Ferrara. "Treatment Decisions in a Skilled Nursing Facility: Discordance with Nurses Preferences." *Journal of the American Geriatrics Society* 33:440 (1985).

3. Bedell, S. E., T. L. Delbanco. "Choices About Cardiopulmonary Resuscitation in the Hospital." *New England Journal of Medicine* 310:1089 (1984).

4. Snow, R. M., K. Atwood. "Probable Death Perspective of the Elderly." *Southern Medical Journal* 78:851 (1985).

6

Rationing of Health Care in Britain: An Ethical Critique of Public Policy-making

John G. Francis
Leslie P. Francis

IN BRITAIN, as in the United States, rationing of health care is a fact of life and death. Some rationing is overt, such as the Stanford heart transplant program's decision not to accept very young or older patients.[1] Some is disguised, such as day-to-day decisions in hospitals about "do not resuscitate" orders[2] or the reported British reluctance to offer dialysis to older patients who might be a bit "crumbly."[3] Some rationing takes the form of absolute barriers to care, such as patient selection criteria. Some involves the refusal to fund care, with the practical result that care is beyond the reach of those who cannot pay. Whether all should have access to at least a decent minimum of health care, and whether rationing can be justified against the background assumption that they should, are complex moral issues, which we shall not tackle directly here.[4] Rather, our aim is to present two factors that are important for the implementation of a rationing policy to be justified, and to explore the extent to which these factors are realized in Britain. Our findings, that Britain falls short of these factors in some glaring ways, yet that rationing occurs, suggest that the rationing that takes place in the National Health Service is not justified at the present time.

First, a word about what we mean by rationing. We use the term very broadly, to include any situation in which distributive issues are taken into account to decide who gets care.[5] Thus, rationing occurs when factors beyond the patient's interests or autonomy are figured into a treatment decision. Common examples of such factors include the patient's age (old or newborn),[6] social status, employment history, ability to pay, and likely life span, or quality of life. To discontinue care that merely prolongs the course of dying, and so will be of limited or no medical benefit, however, is not to ration in the sense with which we are concerned. To be sure, contrasts here are not sharp; quality of life can be so reduced, or life span so abbreviated that it is not in the patient's interests to continue care. The shift to a rationing decision occurs when considerations come into play about how resources could be used elsewhere—when the talk moves to how another patient might make better use of an intensive care unit bed.

Rationing decisions in this broad sense take place all the time. They are adopted as express social policy, such as limits on Medicaid eligibility in the United States, or the British decision to phase in heart and liver transplantation slowly.[7] They take place on the level of individual patient care, too, as when a busy British general practitioner devotes less than five minutes to a patient[8] or an American hospital ethics committee is asked to consider issues in the allocation of hospital resources to patient care.[9]

Justifying Rationing

Whether it occurs on the level of social policy or the level of delivery of care to individual patients, at least two, and perhaps three, factors are important for the rationing of health care to be justified. The importance of these factors is sufficient for our critique of Britain, and we do not make any further claims about whether they are individually necessary or jointly sufficient for rationing to be justified. The factors are, first, that the decision to ration was made with the participation of those whose interests are at stake (or their proxies, if necessary); second, that it was made with awareness that rationing was at issue; and, finally, that those with interests at stake had alternatives available, at least to some limited extent.

These factors are important for several reasons. Access to health care makes a great difference to the opportunities people have, to their ability to live without pain or discomfort, and to life itself.[10] Ill health can strike anyone, even those who take responsible care of their health. If ill health does strike, the financial consequences may be beyond the reach of even the deepest individual pocket or the most prudent individual efforts to buy insurance on the private market.[11]

The randomness of illness and the importance of health care to the quality of life have been taken by some as arguments against rationing health care. In this chapter, we do not draw this inference, but do not thereby mean to suggest it is unjustified. Rather, we take the importance of health care, at minimum, as an argument for the opportunity to participate in a decision to ration. If the decision is to forego care because of its costs, those affected will be the individual patients; if the decision is a matter of social policy, they will be those who gain or lose access to care.

There has been recurring debate in Britain over the adequacy of British political institutions to respond to citizen concerns or to allow affected citizenry to become directly involved in administering programs such as the provision of health care. There are several ways in which such citizen participation might now take place. The traditional view of British political institutions is that Parliament fulfills two critical roles in translating popular preferences into public policy. First, by the doctrine of collective responsibility, the ministers of the government assume complete responsibility for the party's program and performance in office, thus permitting voters to judge, at the time of the general election, their satisfaction or dissatisfaction with the governing party's performance and, at the same time, the merits of the opposition party's proposals. Second, by the doctrine of individual responsibility, the individual minister is held accountable for the actions of his or her ministry's civil servants. According to this doctrine, a misapplication of rules or the abuse of authority by a local health authority is ultimately the responsibility of the minister in charge. Vehicles such as question time enable the members of Parliament to question the appropriate minister about local incidents as though the minister were cognizant of them (although of course he rarely is; nonetheless, he is constitutionally and politically responsible for them). The implication of the doctrine is that serious errors in administration lead to ministerial resignation.

Most commentators writing on the contemporary British constitution would question the extent to which the doctrines of collective and individual responsibility continue to reflect political reality, let alone effectively serve the purpose of legislative oversight. Governments often modify and equivocate on their programs, and few ministers ever resign. Indeed, the doctrine of individual ministerial responsibility may serve to cloak the actions of civil servants, rather than to reveal them to public scrutiny, because questions are directed to ministers and away from civil servants.

The National Health Service (NHS) has not been immune from efforts at reform to find alternative institutional means to achieve greater public scrutiny of and participation in policy-making. One such reform was the 1974 reorganization of the Service, a reorganization that has undergone substantial subsequent modifications. The 1974 reform created fourteen regional authorities responsible for 90 Area Health Authorities, in turn, responsible for 199 District Health Authorities. These areal authorities were created largely to coincide with county boundaries drawn in a then recent local governmental reorganization. A stated goal of the NHS reorganization was to involve many more local authorities in the management of the NHS.

Along with this reorganization of the administrative structure, Community Health Councils (CHCs) were established for each health district. Their membership (of about 30 each) was drawn half from local authorities and half from local voluntary organizations and appointees of the regional Health Authorities. The objective of the CHCs was to represent the public to those who administer the NHS. It appears, however, that few members of the public even know of their existence. The CHCs are strictly advisory in their recommendations and are forbidden to organize nationally. Bates has argued that the CHCs, in spite of not being directly elected, have caused NHS officials to consider the interests of some patient groups that heretofore have been neglected. But Bates does point out that the CHCs cannot or have not been willing "to set priorities for the needs they uncovered and state which services could be reduced to enable the new services to be developed."[12] Most importantly, the efforts at oversight by either Parliament or by citizen bodies have been largely negligible in determining any sort of criteria for the allocation of scarce and expensive medical treatments. As discussed below, these allocative decisions have been the result of central budgetary decisions rather than policy deliberation.

A second factor of importance in the justification of rationing is public knowledge that a rationing decision is at stake. John Rawls has suggested that the requirement that moral principles be public is a "constraint of the concept of right."[13] He makes this suggestion because he believes moral principles are part of a public charter for social life. A community that acts on hidden moral principles lacks a shared moral life—and, not incidentally, is less likely to be one that justifiably claims the loyalty of its citizens.[14] What Rawls does not bring out is the equally important point that those who are left in the dark about the moral principles of their community are, in a sense, second-class citizens. They do not know by what principles their community functions. Not knowing, they will try to change principles with which they disagree. For example, citizens who do not know that their society rations health care, either as a matter of expressed or tacit policy, will not be moved to institute public moral debate on the matter. The practical value of their ability to participate is thereby diminished.

Moreover, those in the dark may easily be victimized by their ignorance. Whether intended or not, one effect of intentional secrecy is to make such victimization easier. No one has to face the pain of an identified victim, because the victims cannot identify themselves. It is much harder to tell a patient with end-stage renal disease that care would help him, but he cannot have it because society refuses to pay, than it is to appear to render a medical judgment that nothing can be done.[15] In rationing situations, it is comfortable to hedge. Hedging, in turn, makes the rationing easier, because no one has to openly face the true anguish of the choice. It also leaves the patient passive, since he does not know that there is any point in even looking for alternatives.

There are certainly a number of ways in which British health care policy can be communicated to the public. Ministerial statements, both in and out of Parliament, convey information. For example, there has been discussion lately of plans to increase the numbers of renal and heart transplants in Britain. Question time in Parliament can be used particularly as a way to air grievances about the impact of policy. The Department of Health and Social Services also issues occasional circulars setting forth policy. What we question below is whether information about policy has been fully articulated, and whether members of the British public have been made sufficiently aware about how policy is translated into practice to appreciate important implications of the translation for individuals' lives. For example, it is one thing to have a publicly-stated policy that the availability of dialysis is based on medical criteria, and another thing to implement financing policies that increase the likelihood that nonmedical factors such as chronological age will play an important role in allocation.

The third factor that makes rationing easier to justify is the availability of alternatives. When scarcity is absolute, it may not be possible to combine a just health care system with full access for everyone to medically feasible alternatives. For example, if the number of transplantable organs is biologically limited, and the supply falls short of needs, a public system of allocation may be the fairest method possible. To allow some private access to suitable organs would be to diminish the public supply.[16] The argument has been made that in any two-tier health care system, the presence of the upper tier threatens to undermine the quality of care available on the basic tier.[17] If there are situations in which the availability of alternatives does not threaten to undermine the quality of basic care, however, such availability makes rationing easier to defend. The individual who loses out on rationed care can seek other sources for care. If such other sources are legally but practically unavailable, most likely because they are too expensive, rationing is correspondingly harder to justify because of the ultimate finality of its effects on lives. If the alternatives are legally prohibited, rationing is harder to justify still to those who have the resources and would choose to purchase care with them. It is perverse comfort to tell such people that they may spend their resources on other luxuries but not on health, especially when their decisions to purchase health would not diminish the resources available to others.

In Britain, for those who can pay for them, alternatives to the NHS are legally available. Private insurance plans fund dialysis, for example. Some organ transplants are funded privately.[18] And the ultimate step of going abroad is always a possibility for those with the means to do so. It should be emphasized, however, that these alternatives are beyond the financial reach of the majority of Britons. Moreover, if British patients are unaware that care is medically possible because allocative decisions are conveyed to them as medical judgments, even available alternatives may be left unexplored.

The NHS: Setting Rationing Policy

The motivating force in the development of the National Health Service was equity in the distribution and provision of medical services. Before the Second World War, there was widespread concern that the state-sponsored health insurance of the Edwardian Liberal governments had not gone far enough in providing health care for the less well off. Enforced migrations to rural areas during the bombings of the Second World War brought home to many Britons the existing sharp geographical differences in medical services and their costs. Some urban areas offered state-assisted medical care at little cost, while most rural areas were without. The war had generated, for many Britons, a strong commitment to equality in the sense that social services—notably health but also housing and education—ought to be made available to all, regardless of station or income.

The overriding concern with equality of access for all to medical services has been apparent throughout the nearly forty years of the Service's operation. Fairly regular investigations are conducted to see if, indeed, treatment has been equitably distributed by class and by region. Yet, there remain significant regional variations in the allocation of resources and persisting sharp differences in life expectations among social classes. For example, British unskilled manual laborers have a two-and-one-half-times greater chance of dying before reaching retirement age than British professionals. Data on self-reported morbidity, particularly chronic illnesses, parallel those on mortality.[19] These inequalities have troubled many proponents of the Health

Service, for whom the core value of the NHS is expressed in the personal experience of one of its most formidable defenders, the late R.M. Titmuss:

> Among all the other experiences I had, another which stands out is that of a young West Indian from Trinidad, aged 25, with cancer of the rectum. His appointment was the same as mine for radium treatments—10 o'clock every day. Sometimes he went into the Theratron Room first, sometimes I did. What determined waiting was quite simply the vagaries of London traffic—not race, religion, colour or class.[20]

The British commitment to equality has been expressed principally in terms of class and geography. Except in some early statements about the importance of the Service to the old and the young, the commitment to equality has not been expressed in terms of age. Class is indirectly related to age in so far as the elderly may be found in greater numbers among the poor. Beyond this indirect relation, however, the NHS has not emphasized age equity, and as we shall see, it appears that age rationing has taken place in practice within the NHS.

The wartime experiences of the population had included rationing of many resources on criteria independent of market allocation. The advocates of state-provided health care argued that medical treatment in postwar Britain should be severed from the marketplace, but delivered more effectively than under the old system. The many government reports that preceded the Act establishing the NHS went beyond treatment of illness by calling for promotion of the positive health of the nation.

The recognition that there would be increasingly hard choices to be made in allocating medical treatment was obscured in the political reality that allowed the National Health Service to come into existence in the postwar years. At that point, the potential—and expense—of medical care to improve life chances seemed likely to lie in better access and in the new wonder drugs, not in capital intensive, extremely expensive therapies. Medicine has, of course, been a rapidly changing field for decades, but what stands out is that many of the advances today are associated with complicated and expensive surgical techniques, in contrast to the 1940s when the emphasis was on new drugs, such as penicillin, that appeared to have vast capacities to cure disease.

What might be described as a second, more recent tradition in the assessment of medicine in Britain has been criticism of the role of technology. British medicine has been faulted for what is described as the undesirable import of American technological medical practices with substantial investment in procedures to prolong life. The criticism is directed to transplants, both organic and mechanical, that seem to absorb significant resources and, in the view of some critics, to overestimate the prolongation of life while undervaluing the quality of life. The 1980 Reith lectures of Ian Kennedy are an example: "The other task doctors in hospitals are performing is that of calling upon more and more complex and expensive technology to respond to situations in which, when one looks at the general overall picture, there is usually little that can be done. To use the metaphor of the mechanic, the tyre can be patched, but even so, it is permanently weak." Kennedy's criticism of technological medicine is combined with a concern that it represents misplaced priorities:

> My second point is that, put baldly, certain services should not be offered until matters of greater priority are dealt with. There are perfectly respectable ethical theories that, in the context of harsh choices such a those we face now (and always as regards resources), allow for conduct that will benefit the larger worthy number even if this inevitably means others may suffer. One example was the decision in the second World War in North Africa that only those who on recovery would be able to fight again should receive scarce penicillin.[21]

This attitude that medicine should provide measured care instead of an all-out onslaught on serious ailments appears to be born out of newer doubts about technology's costs and beliefs in the limits of medical practice. This tradition may, as Aaron and Schwartz suggest,[22] remove some, but by no means all, of the pressure on physicians to engage in expensive procedures.

The great concern for equality and the sense of the limitations of medical treatment are the context in which the National Health Service has operated. Of equal significance to the formation of British health care policy has been the institutional development of the NHS. Until quite recently, the NHS placed the management of health services in the medical community. The compromise that developed between the Labour government of Aneurin Bevan and the British Medical Association during the establishment of the NHS was that doctors would be viewed as independent contractors who would retain autonomy in the performance of their services. In Britain, as in the United States, this is often described in terms of the inviolability of the doctor-patient relationship. By the same token, consultants (as we describe them, specialists) were given control over the administration of hospitals. In effect, a tripartite organization was set up composed of hospital services, community services (local health services), and family practitioner services. In the studies of the NHS, "the National Health Service was bound to be a 'doctor's service' much more than a 'patient's service.' "[23]

Of all the actions of the postwar Labour government, perhaps the most distinctive in organization was granting the medical profession the power to administer the National Health Service. The compromise was probably politically necessary to get the Service established. Nonetheless, the aim of the NHS was medical treatment for all, regardless of condition, and citizen as patient was not given a role in the direction of the NHS save in the form of Parliamentary review.

The 1974 reorganization of the Health Service, described above, was in part motivated by concern to increase participation at the local and lay levels. Local areal authorities were formed to improve coordination in the provision of services. The creation of the Community Health Councils was intended to involve members of the community in assessing the conditions under which medical treatment takes place. In practice, however, the Councils do not seem to have been major consumerist enterprises, but rather to have functioned as organs supporting NHS objectives.[24]

A far more potentially serious institutional modification of the NHS took place eight years later, with the introduction, in 1982, of a management council for the NHS. The Conservative government of the 1980s sought to introduce professional managers and tighter central control over the NHS. They also sought consideration of some forms of privatization in the provision of medical services. The 1982 management reform was seen by the Thatcher government as a crucial step towards cost effective decision-making in the NHS. Some of its apparent implications are discussed below.

Parliamentary review of the NHS has taken the form of the remarkable budgetary control correctly depicted by Aaron and Schwartz. The lid on medical expenditure—although not perhaps as apparent within Britain as it is to students of comparative health care costs—has meant that while the NHS has moved from about 3.2 percent of the GNP to about 5.7 percent in thirty-five years, it remains relatively inexpensive by the standards of other industrialized nations. The pattern in Britain for decades has been limited budgets given to the medical profession to determine, within those parameters, the allocation of resources for medical treatment. This allocation has been complicated more recently by the expense of innovations in medicine both at the diagnostic level and at the level of treatment. In the face of the changing nature of medical practice, the budgetary limitations set by Parliament pose increasing dilemmas for practitioners.

The key qualification of the hope of the NHS in the 1940s to sever the connection between market considerations and medical treatment was the role of the practitioner. In Britain, the need for medical treatment is determined in the first instance of patient care by the general practitioner (GP). The GP performs the central gatekeeping role in the Service by first diagnosing the patient and then determining the type and extent of the treatment (if any) that the patient should receive. Most importantly, the GP determines if the patient should be sent to a consultant or to a hospital for further treatment.

Traditionally, British GPs have made decisions about patient care paternalistically, based on their assessment about what would be best for their patients. Patients are passive and deferential to authority. This passivity may be reinforced by British class structure and attitudes of resignation to illness. It is likely also reinforced by the gatekeeping system itself, under which the GP, not the patient, makes decisions about whether and which specialist to consult.[25] The legal standard in Britain for informed consent to treatment, for example, is what a reasonable physician would disclose; British courts have rejected as inappropriate for British medicine the standard of some American jurisdictions, that the physician must disclose what the reasonable patient would want to know.[26]

The concerns raised by this intersection of GP autonomy and paternalism begin with observation of treatment rates. A survey of disorders with known responsive procedures, found in the population at large in Britain, reveals that patients in Britain ailing from heart and kidney disease or hip problems appear to receive fewer transplants and hip replacements per million than patients in other advanced industrial nations.[27] Within Britain, moreover, there are wide regional and age disparities in rates of treatment.[28]

A central illustration of the dilemma confronting contemporary British medical practice is the introduction of dialysis for the treatment of end stage renal disease. By the early 1970s, British civil servants had become conscious that the new technologies in treatment of renal failure were fairly reliable, lifesaving, and expensive. Rapid advances in medical technology had generated what has been characterized as a "technological imperative." The new procedures were adopted, but incrementally, and it soon became apparent that the United Kingdom's rate of treatment was below that of other nations. The United Kingdom also relied more heavily on less expensive, nonhospital-based therapies such as home dialysis. According to Halper, the low treatment rate falls almost entirely upon those over the age of 45 or suffering complicating diseases.[29]

The willingness of British physicians to accept and work within such a limited program may have reflected a tradition of dealing with limited resources. It is important to emphasize that this tradition antedates the formation of the NHS. British hospitals were in short supply and often seriously outmoded by the 1930s. The war may have reinforced the notion of making do with what was available. Moreover, as Kennedy's Reith lectures seem to imply,[30] physicians coming out of the Second World War may have continued to use the wartime criterion of triage: who can contribute productively to the struggle? Thus, in the 1950s, certain therapies in Britain were given to those who possessed a prior history of gainful employment and seemed likely to continue to work. Rehabilitation services and cataract surgery, for example, were, in the main, restricted to patients under 65.[31] This criterion of social usefulness, if understood in conventional terms, can adversely affect access of the elderly to treatment. It appears inferentially from the distribution of care such as dialysis that such an understanding may have occurred. This understanding is a particular irony since at the outset NHS policy statements had stressed the care of both the elderly and the young.

Halper[32] suggests some additional factors that may have contributed to the informal rationing system that appears to have developed among British physicians. Physicians' committees called to consult with the Ministry of Health about the introduction of dialysis were eager to get the program started and did not question its modest beginnings. The Ministry's interest in cost control coincided with the specialists' emphasis on establishing centers of excellence at major teaching hospitals. When responsibility for funding renal units was turned over to regional health authorities in 1971, it was done within the context of overall financial restrictions. Within this context, general practitioners, who in any event rarely encounter patients with end-stage renal disease, have not developed networks of experience in patient referrals, and may continue to work on outmoded medical assumptions about patient suitability for dialysis. Finally, perhaps because of discouragement and overwork, there are comparatively few nephrologists within the United Kingdom.

The inferential nature of the contention that British physicians employ nonmedical criteria in the allocation of dialysis must be emphasized. Despite the statistics about distribution of treatment, no criteria have been officially articulated by Parliament, the Department of Health and Social Services, or regional or local health authorities on how to allocate treatment for end-stage renal disease. Decisions not to treat those over 45, or those with complicating conditions, have not been made as formal public policy. The dialysis program was established on very limited grounds, and it appears that physicians allocated care within these limits on a more or less informal rationing basis. There is no written policy as to who should receive medical treatment in Britain. Indeed, British writing on health policy suggests an interesting paradox: a good deal of concern for the elderly, but the willingness to resort to an age criterion in times of hard choices.

This paradox may have emerged because the traditional purposes of the Health Service were equality between classes and geographical region, not age cohorts. As we have suggested it also seems likely that institutional structure has played an important role in the apparent resort to age criteria. The preservation of the autonomy of the physician-patient relationship, in the light of limitations on resources, has allowed (or perhaps forced) physicians into establishing their own criteria for determining who is to receive treatment, and physicians appear to have been influenced by triage considerations.

The complexity and risk of the tight budgetary limitations and the failure to articulate criteria for the allocation of health care in a state system are apparent in increasing confrontation between some patient-oriented movements and the NHS. The British Kidney Patient Association (BKPA) claims that between 2000 and 3000 people die yearly from renal failure, and that some portion of these deaths are unnecessary because treatment facilities are too few in number and too unevenly distributed. To dramatize this claim, the BKPA has taken a patient who was refused treatment, and paid for his treatment privately. The Association plans to present the bill to the NHS for reimbursement.

The problem of being refused treatment grows in importance the older a patient becomes; so does the ethical dilemma and the potential legal dilemma faced by physicians. In the view of one commentator, Diana Brahams, the present policy of emphasizing the finite amount of money available and leaving decisions about how to allocate it to local authorities leaves the physician failing in his duty if he tells his patient he is untreatable, when he is indeed treatable but simply not going to be treated because of a lack of facilities. Brahams suggests that the National Health Service Act of 1977 imposes a duty on the Secretary of State for Social Services to provide treatment, and that the failure to treat a treatable patient may allow judicial review and an order for a mandamus to force the Secretary of State to carry out his duty to treat.[33]

Despite efforts by advocacy groups such as the BKPA, it is by no means apparent that we are about to see a significant rise in recourse to the law by British patients. Historically, British patients have not opted for legal action, nor indeed have they employed the NHS-established procedures for complaints. Explanations vary for the limited use of the complaints procedures. Some blame the formality of the procedures for the passivity of patients. It is apparent that while both patient and doctor can elect not to deal with each other and opt for other lists, British patients rarely change physicians except by geographical movement. In effect, the British physician-patient relationship is a remarkably quiescent one in which the patient has come to expect to deal with a single medical authority over the course of much of his or her lifetime. This situation places immense responsibility on the physician, who knows in practice that the patient appears to have no real alternative source of medical advice, and limited prospects for a realistic exit from the medical system. Physician autonomy and Parliamentary cost concerns have interacted in Britain to produce a situation in which this responsibility is not fully exercised on the patient's behalf. Patients, however, may well remain unaware of the failure.

This historical pattern of decision-making for treatment policies in the NHS can surely be criticized. That criticism should not obscure, however, the institutional potential for devising national and explicit criteria for the treatment of patients requiring costly procedures. An illustration of this potential is the Thatcher government's change in NHS managerial strategy. The new strategy is controversial and, indeed, may have been imposed for what might be considered the wrong reasons, to hold steady or cut back health care costs. A national health care management board has been established with an aggressive, interventionist style of national management that seeks to establish efficient health care planning. Day and Klein argue, "The latest round of manpower targets shows that the Department's (Department of Health and Social Service's) long term concern with inputs is undiminished by its more recent interest in outputs."[34]

In large measure, however, the changes in NHS management reflect a new managerial approach in British government. Day and Klein argue that there is an effort for all governmental organizations to have a clear view of their objectives and the means to assess and measure performance in relation to these objectives. Organizations are to have well defined responsibility for making the best use of their resources, particularly money. The NHS, since 1948, has delivered services in response to local priorities of clinicians and health authorities as much as to the explicit directives of central political authorities.

Parliamentary accountability has not really existed for the NHS. The new management plan has potentially sweeping implications for the NHS of imposing a clear sense of national objective. Such a system could establish Parliamentary determination of what the NHS should be about. Presumably, such efforts as the issuance in 1983 of fourteen performance indicators to the fourteen regional authorities and the now 192 local authorities have given the opportunity for national comparisons. This emphasis on performance appraisal could generate pressure to establish differentiated criteria for the allocation of expensive therapies. The driving force for such explicit development of criteria would be to account for sharp regional differentiation in the allocation of therapies at present, and to permit Parliament to come to terms with the de facto criteria for allocation that presently exist. Such a system of national objectives and strict accountability could lead to a sharp departure from the existing system of decentralized autonomy. By contrast, this potential for institutional change is not apparent in the decentralized American system.

The National Health Service was established with the goal of equalizing geographical and class access to medical care. It is ironic that the Service's institutional structure of physician control has discouraged public articulation of treatment goals. The result has been that as the Health Service developed, and costs of treatment increased, physicians have apparently tended to employ implicit rationing criteria. From the data about rates of treatment, it may be inferred that these criteria focus on likely social contribution, and age in particular.

Unfortunately, the use of these criteria was not developed as articulated public policy. To be sure, the increasing concerns of successive Parliament and governments to limit expenditures have been articulated public policy. The problem is not that people in Britain receive fewer hearts *per se*, or indeed, that the political authorities have determined that use of resources to increase such operations is unwise. Our concerns are whether or not there has been an articulation of the criteria actually used in the delivery of health care to British patients, either in the political arena, or on the level of individual patient care. Under the GP gatekeeping system, it is questionable whether knowledge of alternatives is presented to the patient or his designated guardians in a way that allows the opportunity for informed decisions about treatment. How general budgetary limits were to be translated into patient care has been left up to physicians, for the most part. The public, and individual patients, remained relatively unaware that rationing decisions were made because of budgetary limitations. These decisions were especially hard on the elderly. British policy articulated the need to cut health care costs, but did not articulate the bases on which hard choices were to be made.

Recent institutional reforms in the NHS appear to have created a structure within which such allocative criteria can be explicit, publicly responsible policy. Until they become so, however, the age rationing that has developed within the NHS must remain morally suspect. The lesson to be drawn from Britain to the United States is not simply, as Aaron and Schwartz say, that there are hard choices to be made. The other equally important lesson is that it matters institutionally how these choices are made and are communicated to those who must live or die with them.

Notes

1. Shumway now suggests it is medically possible to expand age parameters to below twelve and into, at least, the early 60s. Norman E. Shumway, "Cardiac Replacement in Perspective," *Heart Transplantation* 3:3–5 (1983). The Stanford program's oldest patient to date is in his early sixties.

2. See Steven S. Spencer, " 'Code' or 'No Code': A Nonlegal Opinion," New England Journal of Medicine 300:138–40 (1979).

3. H. Aaron and W. Schwartz, *The Painful Prescription,* Washington, D.C.: Brookings Institution, p. 35 (1984).

4. In a series of recent writings, for example, Norman Daniels argues that age rationing can be justified on prudential grounds. See *Just Health Care,* Cambridge: Cambridge University Press, 1985; "Justice Between Age Groups: Am I My Parents' Keeper?", *Milbank Memorial Fund Quarterly/Health and Society* 61:489 (1983).

5. This is not to equate rationing with any problem of scarcity, but to focus on considerations beyond the individual patient. David Mechanic, for example, characterizes rationing even more broadly then we do, as "no more than a means of apportioning, through some method of allowance, some limited good or service." "Cost Containment and the Quality of Medical Care: Rationing Strategies in an Era of Constrained Resources," *Milbank Memorial Fund Quarterly/Health and Society* 63:453–75, p. 457 (1985).

6. For a good example of the rationing dilemmas posed by the expense of neonatal care, see Tom L. Beauchamp and Laurence B. McCullough, *Medical Ethics: The Moral Responsibilities of Physicians,* Englewood Cliffs, N.J.: Prentice Hall, pp. 146–47 (1984).

7. See Miller, "Reflections on Organ Transplantation in the United Kingdom," *Law, Medicine & Health Care* 13:31–32 (1985). At least part of the delay is also to be attributed to difficulties in obtaining donor organs in Britain.

8. For a description of heavy patient loads of British general practitioners, see Ruth Levitt and Andrew Wall, *The Reorganized National Health Service,* London: Croom Helm, pp. 176–80 (1984).

9. E.g., Hospital Trustee Association of Pennsylvania, "Hospital Biomedical Ethics Committees," *Bioethics Reporter* 3:935 (1984).

10. Norman Daniels, for example, emphasizes opportunity. See Norman Daniels, "Health Care Needs and Distributive Justice," *Philosophy and Public Affairs* 10:146–79 (1981). The other factors may be important in their own right, however, and not simply because they enhance opportunity.

11. Because of their potentially cataclysmic costliness, health care needs are unlike food, housing, and other basic welfare needs. There is, thus, an argument for health insurance, but not for food insurance.

12. Erica M. Bates, *Health Systems and Public Scrutiny, Australia, Britain and the United States,* London: Croom Helm, p. 80 (1983).

13. John Rawls, *A Theory of Justice,* Cambridge: Harvard University Press, p. 133 (1971).

14. This position is not uncontroversial. Calabresi and Bobbitt argue to the contrary that in situations of tragic choice, it may be better for society to dissemble about the decisions being made than to admit openly the devaluation of human life. *Tragic Choices.* New York: W.W. Norton & Co. (1978).

15. In cases in which dialysis turns out to be of problematic benefit, decisions to stop treatment may be more common than is generally recognized. Patients and their families in such situations have a clearer idea of the impact of the therapy on the individual patients involved. It thus may be more reasonable to decide to discontinue treatment, than to refuse, at the outset, to give treatment a try. Neu and Kjellstrand, "Stopping Long-Term Dialysis: An Empirical Study of Withdrawal of Life- Supporting Treatment," *New England Journal of Medicine* 314:14–20 (1986).

16. For a good discussion of one state's efforts to handle this problem, see "Report of the Massachusetts Task Force on Organ Transplantation," *Law, Medicine and Health Care* 13:8–26 (1985).

17. E.g., Amy Gutman, "For and Against Equal Access to Health Care," in President's Commission for the Study of Ethical Problems in Medicine and Biomedical and Behavioral Research, *Securing Access to Health Care,* vol. 2, pp. 51–66 (1983).

18. Miller, "Reflections on Organ Transplantation in the United Kingdom," *Law, Medicine and Health Care* 13:31–32 (1985). Kidney transplants, for example, are performed at the Clementine Churchill Hospital near London, owned by American Medical International, with the kidneys being imported from the United States. Economist Intelligence Unit, *Private Health Care in the United Kingdom: A Review.* London: Economist Publications, p. 41 (1985).

19. "Inequalities in Health," *The Black Report,* Peter Townsend and Nick Davidson, eds. London: Penguin (1981).

20. Brian Abel-Smith and Kay Titmuss, eds., *Social Policy: An Introduction,* London: Allen and Unwin, pp. 150–51 (1974).

21. Ian Kennedy, "Unmasking Medicine," *The Listener,* p. 643 (Nov. 13, 1980).

22. H. Aaron and W. Schwartz, *The Painful Prescription,* Washington, D.C.: The Brookings Institution, (1984).

23. *The English Health Service: Its Origins, Structure and Achievements,* Cambridge, Mass.: Harvard University Press, p. 82 (1958).

24. Erica Bates, *Health Systems and Public Scrutiny, Australia, Britain and the United States,* London and Canberra: Croom Helm (1983).

25. Halper, "End-stage Renal Disease in the United Kingdom," *Milbank Memorial Fund Quarterly/Health and Society* 63:52–93, p. 69 (1985).

26. Schwartz and Grub, "Why Britain Can't Afford Informed Consent," *Hastings Center Report* 15:19–25 (1985).

27. H. Aaron and W. Schwartz, *The Painful Prescription,* Washington, D.C.: The Brookings Institution (1984).

28. Halper, "End-stage Renal Disease in the United Kingdom," *Milbank Memorial Fund Quarterly/Health and Society* 63:52–93, p. 55 (1985).

29. Ibid., p. 55.

30. Ian Kennedy, "Unmasking Medicine," *The Listener* (Nov. 13, 1980).

31. Halper, p. 61.

32. Ibid., pp. 57–59.

33. "End-stage Renal Failure: the Doctor's Duty and the Patient's Right," *The Lancet,* pp. 386–87 (Feb. 18, 1984).

34. Day and Klein, "Central Accountability and Local Decisionmaking: Towards a New NHS," *British Medical Journal,* p. 1676 (June 1, 1985).

Comments

James W. Nickel

I WOULD LIKE TO EXPRESS some concerns about whether the idea of medical rationing is a useful one for our purposes. Second, I will discuss some connections between democratic principles and the justifiability of "rationing" health care.

Is Rationing the Right Concept?

"Rationing" is a dirty word; it suggests shortages, people standing in lines, and unmet needs. Calling what Britain does to contain medical costs "rationing" is likely to lead us to ask how this denial of services can be justified. But, if we rather think of what Britain does as defining the scope of a political right to medical care by seeing what range of claims to services can be met with available resources, then it sounds admirable.

If we are going to use "rationing" as the basis for a philosophical analysis of policy, we need to define it, and this isn't easy—especially if we want to avoid begging fundamental questions. Aaron and Schwartz start with a notion of "full care," which is "all care expected to generate net medical benefits" (*The Painful Prescription*, p. 7). Aaron and Schwartz treat the care received by people in the United States with good health insurance as a working equivalent of this level. Rationing occurs when a level of care, lower than full care, is given in order to save money. The Francises use a somewhat similar approach. They understand rationing to be decisions about medical treatment based wholly or in part by applying a certain kind of rationale or test—one that takes "distributive issues" into account. Distributive issues concern the impact of one patient's treatment on the availability of treatment to others. In a system with a political or insurance-based right to medical services, the alternative to taking distributive issues into account—i.e., engaging in rationing—is providing full care.

Let's go back to the term "full care." First, note the phrase "expected to generate net medical benefits." This assumes that we can distinguish medical benefits from nonmedical benefits, but in order to do so, we will have to appeal to the concept of health. An expansive concept of health will yield an expansive concept of "full care," and this will, in turn, determine what rationing is. Since the notorious vagueness of "health," (and related terms like "recovery"), infects the definition of "full care," it is not surprising that Aaron and Schwartz quickly abandoned their formal definition of full care and simply took what is done for the well insured in the United States as their working criterion.

But taking this level of the best practice in the United States as the norm, and treating levels that fall short of it as rationing, begs a lot of questions. First, it equates technical possibilities (doing everything expected to produce a net benefit) with moral claims, whereas I think that they can only be linked by substantive arguments. Second, it gives at least the appearance of ethnocentrism; it puts the burden of justification on countries that do not do what the United States does for the well insured.

I prefer to see medical care treated like other important, but expensive goods, in that one cannot expect to have a political right to as much as one could conceivably need. A right to education does not include the availability of every educational service from which one could benefit. Similarly, a right to security against crime does not cover every police service that can be expected to provide a security benefit.

Therefore, we need to reject as a norm the medical profession's aspiration to provide everything available, as well as the concept of rationing that it generates. That norm ensures that medical services will be a bottomless pit, and that discussions of appropriate levels of medical service will be dramatized and misinterpreted by being couched as "rationing." Of course, discussions of how much service to provide will still be needed, but they will at least be made easier by the absence of the assumption that we are doing something wrong if we don't provide everything that might help.

Democracy and Medical Rationing

The Francises' criticism of the British National Health Service in terms of democratic principles deserves further comment. This line of criticism reminds us that we should attend, not only to the substantive aspects of the justification of levels of services to be provided, but also to the procedural aspects. Our inquiry needs to include attention to how politically implemented health care systems would need to be chosen and administered to satisfy democratic principles.

We can start, as the Francises do, with the idea that politically implemented health care systems should be selected and receive ongoing scrutiny within a democratic political system. And for this to be a meaningful way for those affected to have a voice in policy, people must know what the system is and what its basic policies are. It is on this point that the Francises are most critical of the British system; they suggest that British medical officials have not been sufficiently forthcoming about the criteria for allocating expensive therapies. "What we question is whether information about policy has been fully articulated, and whether members of the British public have been made aware enough about how policy is translated into practice to appreciate important implications for individuals' lives." Later they say: "The concern is whether or not there has been an articulation of criteria actually used in the delivery of health care to British patients, either in the political arena or on the level of individual patient care. Under the GP gatekeeping system, it is questionable whether knowledge of alternatives is presented to the patient or his designated guardians in a way that gives the patient the opportunity to make informed decisions about his or her next steps, if any."

In discussing dialysis, the Francises make clear that their criticisms include: (1) the failure to formulate and publicize criteria for allocating dialysis; (2) the reliance on general practitioners informally to work out an allocation system; and (3) the resulting lack of information to the public and to patients concerning the availability of dialysis.

The phrase, "articulating a policy," is ambiguous; it can mean either deciding on an explicit policy, or stating that policy so as to make it publicly known. Both senses seem to be part of the criticism that the Francises want to make; they want to criticize British health officials both for failing to decide on a nationwide, explicit policy for limiting levels of services and for failing to inform the public of what that policy is. I will discuss these in reverse order.

Communicating Policies to the Public

Political democracies involve rule by the people, even if that rule is limited to voting for officials and petitioning government. For the people to participate meaningfully through voting and petitioning, they need to have access to information about government actions and policies. We usually speak of this in terms of freedom of information. Some duties of governments, in this regard, are to refrain from lying, obfuscating, or hiding information. This excludes platonic noble lies, coverups, secret actions, and (with some exceptions for military matters) secrecy about actions and policies. Some of the Francises' statements seem to charge that the British government has misled the public: "[I]t is one thing to have a publicly stated policy that the availability of dialysis is based on medical criteria, and another thing to have financing policies in effect that increase the likelihood that nonmedical factors such a chronological age will play an important role in allocation."

Freedom of information also involves duties of officials to communicate general information to the public about actions and policies; these duties may all be discharged by publications (*e.g.*, the *Congressional Record*), hearings, and news conferences. Duties under freedom of information also include good faith response to citizen requests for information about the actions and policies of government agencies. The Francises clearly suggest that the British government has failed in its positive duties to provide information about its policies concerning available medical services. They also seem to suggest that the duty to make information available is especially strong in areas, like medical rationing, where people's lives are at stake.

Deciding on Rationing Policies at the National Level

The Francises also criticize the British government for using decentralized decision-making about allocation, and for leaving decisions about levels of services to be provided to physicians at the local or regional level. The central government has imposed fairly severe budget constraints, and has left it to physicians to restrict services so as to stay within these budgetary limits.

This may be the most controversial of their contentions; it implies that there is something wrong with opting for a decentralized system that leaves fundamental policy decisions to local or regional officials. In dealing with complex problems, contemporary legislatures increasingly allow regulatory and specialized agencies to evolve rules and standards in a piecemeal way. This approach recognizes that legislatures and ministries often lack the knowledge and experience required to formulate workable policies, and allows for flexibility and experimentation at the operations level so that standards can evolve. An official advocating this approach might suggest that working physicians are better positioned than high level officials to know where one can achieve economies while doing the least damage to patient care.

Further, conditions may be very different in different parts of the same country. In a large, remote county with a very low population density, it will be difficult to provide the same levels of patrol or the same response times that are possible in London. Perhaps one could do this if one used helicopters and spent vast sums of money, but this technological possibility falls short of a moral claim. It would be difficult to formulate levels of services in many areas that would be appropriate to both London and these remote counties, and hence one allows officials in these areas to set their own standards with regard to some services. They have the knowledge of what is feasible, given prevailing budgetary levels, that central officials are likely to lack.

A position allowing some decentralized setting of levels of provision is too plausible, in my opinion, to reject wholesale, but several responses are possible. The first recognizes the importance of evolving strategies for economizing at the level of working physicians, but suggests that this process cannot go on forever, that gradually policies should evolve that are judged best and thus applied generally. So although experimentation can occur as one deals with new areas and technologies, formal policies must eventually evolve and be publicized. And here, one can criticize the British National Health System for failing to formalize its policies and communicate them to the public on, for instance, dialysis, where substantial experience has already been acquired.

A second response suggests that flexibility, experimentation, and the accommodation of regional differences—insofar as they imply the absence of publicly known standards—are inappropriate in areas where individuals' lives are at stake. Here, the argument might be that when fundamental human interests and rights are directly jeopardized, higher standards of public scrutiny are appropriate, and hence experimentation and flexibility must be sacrificed if they come into conflict with having clear and publicly known standards. This argument is analogous to one that is often heard in United States constitutional law, namely that an inequality must be subject to stricter judicial scrutiny if it has a substantial impact on fundamental interests or rights. But since a great many medical services have the potential of saving or prolonging life, this argument may protect too much, unless the directness of the connection is made an additional criterion.

7

Artificial Organs, Transplants and Long-Term Care for the Elderly: What's Covered? Who Pays?

Timothy M. Smeeding

Introduction

THERE IS LITTLE ARGUMENT that current health care costs for the elderly are high, and that they will increase by an even greater amount in the future (Meyer 1984; Munnell 1985). Public outlays alone are forecast to rise by 26 percent in real terms (and total health care outlays for the elderly by 23 percent) between 1984 and 2000 due to aging of the population alone, i.e., holding constant health care outlays for age specific subsets of the elderly population and only taking account of increasing numbers of elderly within each age group (Torrey 1985). By 1990 alone, Medicare outlays for the elderly net of covered premiums (for Part B Supplemental Medical Insurance) will reach nearly $100 billion. Moreover, these figures exclude the vast majority of public sector costs of nursing home care (chiefly under the Medicaid program), and other Medicaid and Veteran's Health Care outlays for the elderly. When these expenditures are added in, total public health care expenditures for the elderly are likely to surpass $140 billion in 1990.

Above and beyond the simple effects of aging due to the increased

The author wishes to thank Stephen Long for his most useful comments on an earlier draft of this paper.

longevity of the elderly population over age 65, the growing demand for two particular types of care have the possibility of generating substantially larger increases in health care costs than those forecast above: added outlays for long-term care in nursing home facilities, in community based facilities, or in the home; and Medicare coverage of additional human spare parts—organ transplants and artificial organs.

In evaluating these two types of care and the distribution of their costs and benefits, this paper espouses the broad notion of rationing that Mary Ann Baily (1984) has recently suggested. Rationing involves the process of setting equitable limits on health care availability. This concept of rationing involves a process of emphasizing equity in the face of scarcity. In other words, if one thinks that health care resources should be allocated in accord with an equity principle, e.g., that the rich pay a higher share of their incomes for care than the poor, we feel that this involves rationing. We wish, then, to address the issue of the health care rationing among the elderly from two policy perspectives: (a) Which medical procedures should be "entitled," should qualify for publicly financed provision of care? and (b) How might the costs of providing publicly financed (and other) health care be shared more equitably among elderly health care recipients, their families, and taxpayers?

To be sure, these questions are related and involve principles of both ethics and economics. While economists wear no special mantle in the ethics arena, one thoughtful economist (Thurow 1984: 1569–1570) neatly summarized the dilemma as follows:

> Ethically, most Americans are simultaneously egalitarians and capitalists. None of us wants to die because we cannot afford to buy medical care, and as egalitarians few of us want to see others die because they cannot afford to buy medical care. As capitalists, Americans believe that individuals should be allowed to spend their money on whatever they wish, including health care.
>
> This set of beliefs leads to an explosive chain reaction. A new expensive treatment is developed. In accordance with capitalistic principles, the wealthy are allowed to buy the treatment privately regardless of its medical effectiveness. Persons with a moderate or low income who cannot privately afford the treatment want it. They demand it. Being egalitarians, Americans do not have the political ability to say "no" to any person dying from a treatable disease. Ways are found to provide the treatment through private or public health insurance. Being egalitarians, we have to give the treatment to everyone or deny it to everyone; being capitalists, we cannot deny it to those who can afford it. But since resources are limited, we cannot afford to give it to everyone either.

Short of increasing health care costs to 15 percent (or more) of the national product (Binstock 1985), is there any way out of this conundrum? Can or should we come to some moral agreement on how to say no as far as the public purse strings are concerned? The answer, I think, is yes. This answer involves the two basic health care rationing steps suggested above: first, deciding what should be covered by public health insurance for the elderly; and second, deciding who should pay for the public (and other) costs of that care.

Rationing of health care is not a novel idea. Rationing deals generally with the way in which health care is distributed (Fuchs 1984; Francis and Francis 1985). We ration (distribute) health care all the time: by entitlement (to private or public insurance); by queue (in the case of most types of organ transplants and other procedures where demand exceeds supply); by third party decision (e.g., relatives, courts of law, hospital review boards); and perhaps, most of all, by willingness and ability to pay (since entitlement to high quality medical care and access to organ transplants is positively correlated with wealth, income, and social position by all of which we mean ability to pay). The question that needs to be addressed then is how much weight to put on each of these rationing devices? Although this chapter deals only with two of these—entitlement and ability to pay—it probably deals with the two most important rationing devices for health care.[1] For purposes of this chapter, entitlement is synonymous with pubic insurance (Medicare and Medicaid) coverage of a particular health care procedure. In order to illustrate these principles, two examples of costly health care entitlements are used: entitlement to human spare parts (transplants), and entitlement to long-term care under the Medicare program.

In the next section, I will outline the methods by which economists might determine entitlement via public sector coverage for these procedures. The third section deals with who should pay for this coverage, and the fourth with policy alternatives to deal equitably with the cost of financing health care for the elderly.

How Should Entitlement to Public Health Care Procedures be Rationed?

The economists' answer to determining entitlement for health care procedures is straightforward. At the very least, we need to decide whether the health outlays are going to be cost-beneficial (i.e., are the benefits going to outweigh the costs) as a necessary condition; and secondly, are these outlays more or less cost-beneficial than alternative uses of the same funds, as a secondary condition? Rational public resource allocation in health care, national defense, and education suggest that both criteria, necessity and sufficiency, be addressed in

determining health care coverage for public programs. Unfortunately, in the case of health care, cost-benefit analysis involves
estimating the value of human life as a measure of the benefit of
health care outlays and, because human life is not a marketed good,
our methods for measuring such benefits are fairly crude at this time
(e.g., see Landefeld and Seskin 1982; Avorn 1984). If we limit ourselves instead to allocation of public resources within health care
programs alone, and if we assume that the goal of these outlays is to
provide the largest number of high quality life years as a benefit per
dollar of health care outlay, tcost-effectiveness analysis can be substi-
tuted for cost-benefit analysis.

The nuts, bolts, promises, and pitfalls of cost-effectiveness analysis
in health care have been aptly demonstrated by others, and will not
be repeated here (e.g., see Weinstein and Stason 1978; Smeeding and
Straub 1984; Warner and Luce 1982). Rather, our purpose is to simply
illustrate the implications of cost-effectiveness analysis for health care
entitlement among the elderly as compared to other groups in society. The logic and, therefore, the answer is straightforward: health
care procedures are likely to cost more for the elderly than for other
groups simply because of the generally lower health status of the
elderly, while the benefits are liable to be lower because the expected
improvement in quantity (years) and quality of life is lower than for
other groups. The lesser health status (lower quality of remaining life)
is largely due to chronic health conditions (arthritis, hypertension,
etc.) among those age 65 and over as compared to the younger
population (National Center for Health Statistics 1983). While physical frailty cannot be generalized to all persons at any given age, and
while there is nothing magical about age 65 (other than its general use
to separate the elderly from the rest of the population and to obtain
Medicare coverage), it seems clear that the necessary conditions for a
medical procedure to become cost-effective are more likely to be met
among younger as compared to older persons. It is important to note
that this is quite simply the result of applying generally accepted
criteria to health care procedures for persons of different ages. To call
the result "age discrimination" (Avorn 1984) is to deny the general
usefulness of the criteria itself. The case of major organ transplants
may help clarify the way in which these criteria might be applied in
determining rationing of health care entitlement between the elderly
and others in society.

Spare Parts

Organ transplants and artificial organs are proving cost effective
under conditional entitlement criteria for some groups of both de-
manders and suppliers. For persons in otherwise good health, and

for medical care suppliers sufficiently staffed, qualified, and experienced to provide a particular type of organ transplant, the outcome can be quite positive. Over 90 percent of all transplants are for kidneys that are of fairly low cost ($40,000), particularly when compared to dialysis, that is of high benefit, particularly among children (Iglehart 1984). Kidneys are much cheaper than heart ($100,000) or liver ($135,000) transplants, but even heart transplants are now proving cost effective under the best clinical and patient circumstances (see Auten and Cosimi 1984; EBRI 1984; and Evans 1982). While data on more widespread provision and full blown cost-benefit analyses of transplants at multiple sites still need to be made, many private insurance carriers and some public programs (e.g., Blue Cross in Massachusetts, Medicaid in Maryland and in some other states) have moved heart transplantation from an uncovered "experimental procedure" to a covered "therapeutic procedure." But by and large, these programs do not cover elderly persons. The question of whether or not Medicare should move to cover heart or liver transplants as a therapeutic procedure for the elderly has not yet been answered.

Currently, the Medicare program pays for some less expensive nonrenal transplants (cornea, skin), and for some artificial organs (hip or joint replacement). These are generally accepted to be cost-effective. But what of heart and liver transplants? The most successful heart transplantation programming the United States (and probably in the world) at Stanford University just recently extended its upper age range of eligibility to 55 and is considering expanding to age 60 (Shumway 1983). Congressman Gore has sponsored legislation (HR 4080) that would permit Medicare funded heart transplantation in limited numbers of cases. But to date, there has been little or no experience with heart transplantation among those age 65 (Medicare qualification point for the nondisabled) or older. In fact, the world's first two artificial heart recipients (Clark and Schroeder) were refused heart transplants at Stanford because they were beyond the age cutoff. Liver transplantation is much the same. In the United States, they are generally limited to young children born with malfunctioning livers (Meyer 1984); there is no experience with liver transplantation among persons age 50 or older anywhere in the world (Caplan 1983).

Certainly, the demand for transplanted hearts and livers among the elderly abounds. About 40,000 adults (mainly with cirrhotic livers) could benefit from a liver transplant.[2] About 10,000 or more of these are Medicare eligible. In a study on the artificial heart commissioned by Congress, 70 percent of the viable candidates for heart transplantation in 1979, about 80,000 persons, were age 65 or over

(Lubeck and Bunker 1982). Estimates of the 1984 cost of such procedures range from $12 to $20 billion (Meyer 1984 and author's arithmetic). But studies of those who could *potentially* benefit from transplantation must be carefully separated from those whereby transplantation could prove cost-effective. For instance, of the 112,000 or more persons (including the 80,000 elderly) who might benefit from an artificial heart (Lubeck and Bunker 1982), only about 3000-5000 meet the strict (and cost-effective) eligibility criteria that the Stanford program has established (Austin and Cosimi 1984). Most fail on age grounds, but at least 25,000 persons under age 65 who would benefit from a heart transplant do without.

The reason for rationing heart and liver transplants to these groups is, in one sense, straightforward: limited supply. But behind the limitations of supply are social and medical judgments indicating toward whom these life extending procedures should be directed, even in an experimental sense. The elderly were not among those chosen for either program, perhaps because the implicit cost-effectiveness standards that underlie the eligibility criteria for heart and liver transplants indicated that younger patients should be treated first.

But now, as heart transplantation begins to move beyond its experimental stage, and as efforts to expand the supply of human organs and artificial organs (a temporary, if not a permanent, substitute for a human organ) increase, we should face the problem of Medicare entitlement for transplantation head on. Already, we have made the decision to proceed with the development of the artificial heart, and while early experimentation is not terribly encouraging, it seems unwise to deny continued experimentation. A recent study commissioned by the National Heart, Lung, and Blood Institute (1985) forecasts that within 15 years a fully implantable heart could provide a significant increase in life span for up to 35,000 persons age 70 and under each year. The total cost of implantation alone would be about $5.3 billion.

If a bill such as HR 4080 allows for even limited, conditional, selective Medicare payment for heart transplants or artificial hearts, these funds should be used to provide some evidence of the relative cost effectiveness of such procedures for the elderly before it becomes general Medicare policy to entitle anyone to heart or liver transplantation. If properly put to use, such data would allow certain procedures and transplants to be classified as efficacious, therapeutic, and cost-effective for some groups, while still experimental and unproven for others. At the very least, we must experiment with transplants for older persons before we entitle them to coverage. While HR 4080 still awaits passage, a modest beginning towards providing the data on organ procurement, distribution, and efficacy of transplantation needed to make such an assessment has been made with passage of the Hatch Bill (S 2048) in late 1984, which created a task force to study organ transplantation issues.

Long-Term Care

Another example of a potentially costly but also potentially cost-beneficial public outlay largely for elderly persons is the issue of long-term care outlays. In the United States today, long-term care is provided in three general types of facilities: skilled nursing homes (or intermediate care facilities); smaller congregate facilities (largely experimental); and in the home, either formally (via publicly supported home health care), or informally (via unpaid care provided by relatives or friends). For the most part, long-term care is provided informally by relatives or friends. Medicare coverage of skilled nursing care is limited both in amount of outlay per day and in length of coverage such that only about three percent of Medicare Part A outlays (about $.7 billion in 1984) went for "long"-term care. In fact, the current logic behind Medicare payments for these programs is more akin to supporting short-term institutional substitutes for hospitalization than long-term care *per se*. About half of all direct payments for long-term care (about $1 billion) are paid for by public programs, and the very large majority of these funds (90 percent) come from the Medicaid program. The major question to be addressed here is, should Medicare move to provide entitlement to truly long-term care on a permanent basis?

There has been very little cost-benefit or cost-effectiveness analysis of long-term care as a medical procedure. One reason is that much of long-term care funds are *not* for medical care at all, but are for the basic necessities of life: food and shelter. Thus, it may be wrong to classify long-term care as health care in the usual sense of the word. Secondly, long-term Medicare deals with a different type of health care. In many cases, the needs of long-term care beneficiaries arise from chronic, not immediately life-threatening, health care problems resulting in need for assistance in rehabilitative exercise, eating, walking, cleaning, and continency. In fact, life saving and/or life extending medical care decisions for the elderly in long-term care are, by and large, made by the same persons (doctors, family, and other providers) in the same setting (hospitals) as for the noninstitutionalized elderly. Thus, it may not be wise to apply medical cost-effectiveness analysis to the chronic health care needs of this population in the same way that we apply it to medical procedures such as artificial organs.

The cost per case of providing long-term care for any given person can be quite different in an institutional setting (e.g., nursing home) as compared to long-term care in one's own home, because: (1) the latter necessarily entails implicit provision of food and shelter; and (2) because quite often the elderly patient has needs less than the full range of services offered in a skilled nursing facility. In many cases, home health care can be provided at lower cost per case than can institution-based care. The cost problem with moving to "less expensive" home health care on a permanent Medicare funded basis is twofold: (1) the number of potential home health care beneficiaries is much larger than the number of those needing and receiving institution-based long-term care; and (2) the decision of who should pay for long-term care: the elderly, their families, or the public, needs to be answered before such entitlement is granted. In this case, as perhaps also with the case of the transplant, the question of public program eligibility or rationing of long-term care is really a question of who should pay for care: the public (via tax and transfer programs), or the recipients and, either explicitly or implicitly, their families? Were Medicare to begin to fund long-term home, community, or institution-based care on a permanent basis, public long-term care outlays would increase by at least $10 billion per year. Already, there are at least twice as many persons not in nursing homes who are as chronically disabled as those in nursing homes, in terms of limited daily activities, and perhaps as many as five times that number (George 1985). This need is most apparent among the oldest of the elderly. For instance, of the home based population age 85 or over, 43 percent needed help in one or more basic activities in 1979-1980, while more than 20 percent of the population age 85 and over resided in nursing homes in 1980 (U.S. Senate 1984; Feller 1983). Thus, the question of who should pay for long-term car looms large as a public policy rationing issue. We now turn to the question of who should pay.

Who Pays?

Heavily involved in the issue of coverage for transplantation, for long-term care and for other health care needs, is the question of financial liability for health care for the elderly. One might successfully argue that medical procedures that meet cost-effectiveness criteria should be provided by public entitlement. But entitlement alone does not answer the question, who should pay for these public entitlement programs? Medical procedures that have not met cost-effectiveness criteria and that remain in an experimental phase are likely to be rationed on the basis of ability to pay, even, if formally, they are rationed by other means (e,g., queues). Also, medical care services only partially covered by public programs are otherwise paid for by recipients or by other third parties. But should public programs be financed according to ability to pay as well? To begin to answer this question, it seems important to establish ability to pay among groups and individuals in society. Within this realm it is necessary to realize that many of the elderly do indeed have the ability to pay for their own health care whether by means of public programs such as Medicare, by means of private health insurance, or by direct payment.

Ability to Pay for Acute Care

The high average absolute and relative (to the younger population) level of economic well-being among the elderly in the United States has been reasonably well established (Danziger, et al. 1982; Smeeding 1985). Relatively few elderly fall below the official United States poverty line (U.S. Bureau of the Census 1985; Smeeding 1982). Further, the elderly are no more nor less vulnerable to inflation than are any other groups in the population—they do *not*, by and large, live on "fixed incomes" (Hurd and Shoven 1984; Clark et al. 1982). There is also recent evidence that the elderly do not decumulate their substantial assets as they age (Menchik and David 1983), and that among all population age groups, the elderly experienced the largest increase in real income between 1979 and 1984 (Palmer and Sawhill 1984). Taking into account differences in household size and composition, taxes, and income in kind from public transfers, employment related benefits, and housing, the economic status of the elderly as a group is 10 to 15 percent higher than that of the nonelderly (Smeeding 1985).

However, this conclusion needs to be tempered by two additional observations concerning single elderly females (and males) over age 75—the group most likely to be in need of long-term care. First of all, as the elderly grow older, their relative economic status diminishes (Duncan, Hill, and Rodgers 1985; Smeeding 1985). For instance, single females age 75 or older are only about 75–85 percent as economically well off as those under 65, all things considered, while elderly couples age 65–70 are much better off. Secondly, within every age group of the elderly, there is considerable diversity in economic status, or as economists would say, large variance around the mean (Quinn 1984). While single elderly females are on the average not very well off, many of them are still relatively well off. More than 30 percent had cash incomes at least twice a great as the amount defined as poverty (about $12,000) in 1983. While separate data on single females age 75 or older is difficult to obtain, according to a 1979 survey over half of those families headed by a person age 75 or over had liquid assets of $30,000 or more, while 30 percent had more than $50,000 (Radner and Vaughn 1983). Families headed by a person age 75 or older also had net financial assets as large as all those age 65 to 74 (Radner 1984). Futhermore, 59 percent of the elderly owned homes with an average net worth of $33,000 (Torrey 1985). Thus, a sizeable minority of families and persons age 75 or over have some ability to pay for their own health care. But on the other hand, many do not. Medical needs increase among the oldest old at the same time that income, assets, and ability to pay diminish (Atkins 1985). While these data indicate that economic justice in allocation of health care resources should be independent of age (Binstock 1985), great care needs to be taken in measuring financial ability to pay for health care needs. The current way in which we pay for health care and health care entitlement programs for the elderly is instructive in this regard.

Medical ability to pay can be somewhat different than overall economic status.[3] Here, it is not only income but also entitlement to Medicare and nonMedicare health insurance coverage that determines who will pay for medical care for the elderly. For instance, consider serious medical illnesses other than long-term care, *e.g.*, the types of situations where organ transplants might be most often in demand. In such cases, Medicare coverage alone is hardly sufficient to forestall economic catastrophe. In 1979, Medicare on the average covered only about 60 percent of the health care costs of its noninstitutionalized elderly enrollees. Among the 19.5 million elderly Medicare enrollees in 1979, 58 percent had only Medicare as *subsidized* health care coverage. (Many of these purchased a supplemental "medigap" policy to complement Medicare, but they purchased it out of their own funds.) The other 42 percent had at least one additional health insurance source paid for by a third party: the government via Medicaid or Veteran's Health Care for two-thirds of these, and a current or former employer or union for the other third. The 58 percent who had only Medicare paid just over 40 percent of their health expenses out of pocket either directly or by purchasing private "medigap" health insurance policies that supplemented their Medicare coverage. Within this group with only Medicare as subsidized coverage, 43 percent had money incomes between the poverty line and twice the poverty line (about $5200–$10,400) in 1979. For this 24 percent of all elderly persons, out-of-pocket expenses averaged 19 percent of money income with a wide variance in expenses within this group. Many of the elderly poor with substantial medical care needs had Medicaid to supplement their Medicare coverage,[4] while most of those above twice the poverty line were either subsidized by employers or could well afford medigap coverage. The 43 percent with only Medicare as subsidized coverage, who fall in between Medicaid poor and the well-to-do, are in serious risk of medical economic disaster. While they are economically better off than their Medicaid eligible peers, they do not enjoy anywhere near the same level and type of health care protection as do the poor.

Ability to Pay for Long-Term Care

The case of ability to pay for nursing home or other long-term care expenditures is very different. Other than Medicaid, there is virtually no widespread institutional mechanism to insure against the substantial costs of long-term care, which averaged $2200 per month in 1984. Most nursing home residents are female (70 percent), with an average age at first admission of 80, usually following hospitalization. Most enter under their own financial resources and/or in combination with Medicare. Many of these who enter under their own finances (estimates range between 35 and 45 percent) end up spending themselves into penury, at which point Medicaid takes over. Others die before their financial resources are exhausted. Interestingly, children are not legally liable for supporting the long-term care needs of parents, regardless of the child's economic well-being. Yet, nursing homes are, to a large extent, the inventions of children. Were it not for these institutions, the adult children of the elderly would be the ones to provide aid, either financially or by directly providing long-term care in kind by taking care of their parents (Lampman and Smeeding 1983). As we deliberate the question of who should pay for the long-term care needs of the elderly, these indirect beneficiaries of public programs should be considered as well.

Policy Implications

Health care needs and ability to pay for those needs are often at odds among the elderly and among other groups as well. One way to provide financial assurance in case of medical needs is via entitlement to public programs. Medicare covers virtually all of the elderly, but pays only about 60 percent of the costs of health care for noninstitutionalized coverees. Only the poor elderly (Medicaid), and some elderly male veterans (Veteran's Health Care) have other public subsidies for noninstitutional health care costs. Increasingly financial public pressures are leading to reductions in Medicare (and Medicaid) outlays via higher coinsurance or deductibles and lower payments to suppliers (physician fee scales and prospective reimbursement).

These cutbacks will provide increased pressure on nonMedicare sources for health care coverage. Who should cover these costs?

Against this background of fiscal restraint, a growing elderly population and new medical procedures, e.g., major (heart, liver) organ transplants, are generating increased demand for more and better coverage, including coverage of long-term care by non-means tested public programs such as Medicare. Faced with this dilemma, and in light of a large federal budget deficit,[5] policymakers have, for the most part, indicated a willingness to reduce health care outlays in only a simplistic, across-the-board fashion. But fiscal ability to pay should not be the way that health care is rationed among the elderly in America. Principles of cost effectiveness and individual ability to pay should govern what public programs will cover for the elderly and also who should pay for these covered health care services.

First of all, we need more and better data on the health outcomes and costs of heart and liver transplants or artificial organ substitutes for the elderly before they become generally accepted treatments. Until that evidence has been gathered, it is not advisable to extend Medicare coverage to these medical procedures. If and when it can be shown that such programs are cost effective, public entitlement should be extended to all who are in need. Until that time has come, only the rich (or others) who are willing to pay for experimental treatments should be afforded that coverage and only when more qualified candidates, e.g., those who are generally younger and healthier, have been treated first.

Even if expensive health care treatments are made available on an entitlement basis to the elderly on cost-effectiveness grounds, public policy still needs to address the issue of the distribution of payment for noninstitutional health care treatment more effectively than is currently the case. Ability to pay should be free from age bounds: the elderly who can well afford to cover a greater share of their health care expenses should do so, and those who are only marginally able to provide for themselves should be given greater financial relief, regardless of age.

One promising alternative to reaching both of these goals is an expansion of Medicare to cover a greater range of potential health care costs, with this expansion financed by an income-related premium paid for by the elderly themselves (Davis and Rowland 1984). Such a program might require consolidation of Medicare and Medicaid for the elderly and would promise a more equitable distribution of the burden of medical expenses. Currently, the elderly premiums for Medicare are about $200 per year. These supplemental medical insurance premiums cover only about 25 percent of Medicare Part B

costs or 9 percent of total programs outlays (Munnell 1985). The rest
are paid from payroll and income taxes largely levied on the younger
population. These premiums are not income scaled and there is no
premium for Part A, hospital coverage. An income-related premium
for Medicare, Parts A and B combined, would provide a more rational
method of payment for health care entitlements among the Medicare
population, a payment based on insurance costs rather than on
medical needs, and a payment that would more fairly share these
health care costs between generations.[6] Moreover, such a changeover
might allow limited additional financial support for currently non-
Medicaid eligible low-income individuals age 60 or over who do not
qualify for publicly provided health care as disabled individuals.

In the case of long-term care, the current system is a good beginning. However, for those who wish to avoid the high risks of financial
disaster and subsequent reliance on Medicaid, new efforts to offer
public and private long-term-care insurance on a voluntary basis
must be made. Prototypical long-term-care policies have been developed and appear quite reasonable for both institutional and home
care settings *if* purchased at an early enough age (Meiner and Trapnell
1984). Public efforts to subsidize such coverage via tax avoidance
mechanisms for long-term-care premiums are one way to induce
demand for these programs. Employers may find it to their advantage
to offer private long-term-care insurance as a benefit to older workers
and recent retirees. If employers and private insurance agencies are
not willing to offer such coverage on a wide scale basis, perhaps the
federal government should consider it as an optional part of Medicare
coverage, with a separate premium. Such developments would offer
tomorrow's elderly the choice of insuring now or running the financial risk of penury (to qualify for Medicaid coverage) at a later time.
Right now only the second choice is available.

Another possibility is to directly tap the incomes of the children of
the low-income institutionalized elderly to cover the costs of their
parents' care on an ability to pay basis. Such a scheme was temporar-
ily enforced in Idaho in 1984, but was later declared illegal. On ethical
grounds, a case can be made for children helping to support their
parents in such instances. However, a federal public policy in this
arena has not yet been forthcoming.[7]

Conclusion

In a recent report to the Health Insurance Association of America,
based on 125 interviews with leading health care professionals (physicians, academics, insurers, business and labor leaders), Arthur D.
Little, Incorporated (1984) predicted a two-tier system of health care

in the United States by 1995. Certain groups (the poor, the underinsured) would receive a different type and quality health care as compared to the wealthy and the heavily insured. Health care for all would not be equal in either quality or quantity.

This chapter speaks to this scenario by suggesting that certain treatments that are not proven cost-effective *should be* rationed largely by ability to pay. If so, the elderly with enough resources to cover such treatments as heart or liver transplants will be able to afford them. It seems that this type of two-tier health care system might be acceptable and even desirable considering rational allocation of public health care resources.

However, we should be able to do a better job of providing effective and necessary medical care to the elderly by developing a more rational and equitable means of paying for that care. To the extent that we can tap the resources of the elderly themselves, or their children, via either greater reliance on income related premiums for medical procedures or alternative voluntary insurance arrangements for long-term care, we may be able to avoid the negative consequences of a two-tier health care system for the elderly.

Instead of simplistic budget-cutting exercises in the Medicare-Medicaid long-term-care arena, perhaps it is time for the federal government to positively approach the issue of health care entitlements and payment mechanisms for the elderly. It seems that we should do something before the health care provider industry marches elderly hypertensives and end-stage coronary disease cases into a congressional hearing carrying their artificial hearts and pleading for their lives. We can and should do a better job of rationing health care among the elderly in the United States.

References

Atkins, G. 1985. "The Economic Status of the Oldest Old." *Milbank Memorial Fund Quarterly/Health and Society,* vol. 63, no. 2:395–419.

Austen, W. G. and A. B. Cosimi. 1984. "Heart Transplantation After Sixteen Years." *New England Journal of Medicine,* vol. 311, no. 22. (November 29):1436–1438.

Avorn, J. 1984. "Benefit Cost Analysis in Geriatric Care: Turning Age Discrimination Into Health Policy." *New England Journal of Medicine,* vol. 310, no. 20. (May 17):1294–1301.

Baily, M. A. 1984. "Rationing and American Health Policy." *Journal of Health Politics, Policy and Law,* vol. 9, no. 3 (Fall):489–501.

Binstock. R. H. 1985. "The Oldest Old: A Fresh Perspective or Compassionate Ageism Revisited?" *Milbank Memorial Fund Quarterly/Health and Society,* vol. 63, no. 2:420–51.

Caplan, A. 1983. "Organ Transplants: The Costs of Success." *Hastings Center Report,* vol. 13, no. 6 (December):23–32.

Clark, R. et al. 1982. "Inflation and Economic Well-Being of the Elderly." Final Report, National Institute on Aging. September.

Danziger, S. et al. 1982. "Income Transfers and the Economic Status of the Elderly." Institute for Research on Poverty Discussion Paper #695-82, University of Wisconsin, Madison. July.

Davis, D., D. Rowland. 1984. "Medicare Financing Reform: A New Medicare Premium." *Milbank Memorial Fund Quarterly/Health and Society*, vol. 62, no. 2:300–16.

Duncan, G., M. Hill, W. Rodgers. 1985. "The Changing Economic Status of the Young and Old." Prepared for the National Academy of Sciences Workshop on Demographic Change and the Well-Being of Dependents. July 18.

Employee Benefit Research Institute. 1984. "Rationing the High Cost of Health Care: The Case of Organ Transplants." Washington: Employee Benefit Research Institute Issue Brief #31. June.

Evans, R. 1982. "Economic and Social Costs of Heart Transplantation." *Heart Transplant 1982*, vol. 1:243–51.

Feller, B. A. 1983. "Americans Need Help to Function at Home." *Vital and Health Statistics*, no. 92, National Center for Health Statistics. September 14.

Francis, L. and J. Francis. 1985. "The Rationing of Health Care in Britain: An Ethical Critique of Public Policymakers." Prepared for the Utah Conference on Health Care Rationing among the Elderly. September 13.

George, L. 1983. "A Review of Evidence of Family Support for Older Persons." Presented to the National Academy of Sciences Workshop on Demographic Change and the Well-Being of Children and the Elderly. September 5.

Hurd, M., J. Shoven. 1984. "Inflation Vulnerability, Income and Wealth of the Elderly, 1969–1979." Forthcoming in M. David and T. Smeeding, eds., *Horizontal Equity, Uncertainty, and Economic Well-Being*. National Bureau of Economic Research Conference on Research in Income and Wealth, vol. 50 (Chicago: University of Chicago Press).

Lampman, R. and T. Smeeding. 1983. "Interfamily Transfers as Alternative to Government Transfers to Pensions." *Review of Income and Wealth*. March.

Landefeld, J. S. and E. P. Seskin. 1982. "The Economic Value of Life: Linking Theory to Practice." *American Journal of Public Health*, vol. 72, no. 6:555–56.

Little, A. R., Inc. 1984. "The American Health Care System in 1995." Prepared for the Health Insurance Association of America.

Lubeck, D. and J. Bunker. 1982. "The Artificial Heart: Cost, Risks, and Benefits." Case study #9, for background paper #2, Case Studies of Medical Technologies for the Office of Technology Assessment. May.

Meiners and Trapnell. 1984. "Long Term Care Insurance, Premium Estimates for Prototype Policies." *Medical Care*, vol. 22, no. 10: 901–11.

Menchik, P., M. David. 1983. "Income Distribution, Lifetime Savings and Bequests." *American Economic Review*, 73–77. September:672–90.

Meyer, J. 1984. "Implications of Aging Populations for Health Care Policy and Expenditure." For the Working Party on Social Policy. Office of Economic Cooperation and Development. Paper MAS/WP1(84)3. Paris: 24 September.

Munnell, A. 1985. "Paying for the Medicare Program." *New England Economic Review*. Jan./Feb.:47–61.

National Center for Health Statistics. 1983. *1981 National Ambulatory Medical Care Survey*. Unpublished data.

National Heart, Lung and Blood Institute. 1985. "Artificial Heart and Assist Devices: Directions, Needs, Costs, Societal and Ethical Issues." Presented to the National Advisory Council of the National Heart, Lung and Blood Institute. May.

Palmer, J. and I. Sawhill, eds. 1984. *The Reagan Record*. Urban Institute Book. (Cambridge: Ballinger). August.

Quinn, J. 1984. "The Economic Status of the Elderly: Beware of the Mean." Mimeo. Chestnut Hill. Boston College. October.

Radner, D. 1984. "The Wealth and Income of Aged Households." Presented to the American Statistical Association. August.

Radner, D. and D. Vaughn. 1983. "The Joint Distribution of Wealth and Income for Age Groups." Prepared for the C.V. Starr Conference at New York University, November 10, 1979. Mimeo.

Shumway, N. 1983. "Cardiac Replacement in Perspective." *Heart Transplant* 3:3–5.

Smeeding, T. and L. Straub. 1984. *"Health Care Financing Among the Elderly: the Medicare Crisis."* Prepared for the 6th Annual Meeting of the Association for Public Policy Analysis and Management, New Orleans. October.

Smeeding, T. 1982. *Alternative Methods for Valuing Selected In–Kind Transfers and Measuring Their Impact on Poverty.* U.S. Bureau of the Census. Technical Report #50. April.
———. 1985. "Full Income Estimates of the Relative Well-Being of the Elderly and the Nonelderly." Final report for contract #UAD 935W712, to the Institute for Research on Poverty, University of Wisconsin, Madison. Mimeo. May.
Thurow, L.C. 1984. "Learning to Say 'No'." *New England Journal of Medicine,* vol. 311, no. 24 (December 13):1569–1572.
Torrey, B. 1985. "Sharing Increasing Costs on Declining Income: The Visible Dilemma of the Invisible Aged." *Milbank Memorial Funding Quarterly/Health and Society,* vol. 63, no. 2:377–94.
U.S. Bureau of the Census. 1985. "Money Income and Poverty Status of Families and Persons in the United States: 1984." *Current Population Reports,* series P-60, no. 148. (Washington, U.S. Government Printing Office). August.
U.S. Senate. 1984. *Aging America: Trends and Projections by the Special Committee on Aging.* U.S. Senate. May.
Warner, K. and B. Luce. 1982. *Cost-Benefit and Cost-Effectiveness Analysis in Health Care.* Ann Arbor: University of Michigan Press.
Weinstein, M. and N. Stason. 1978. "Foundations of Cost-Effectiveness Analysis for Health and Medical Practices." *New England Journal of Medicine* 305 (March 31):716–53.

Notes

1. In cases where demand exceeds supply, one's position in the queue is often determined, implicitly or explicitly (blackmarket), by ability to pay. For instance, recent covert activities related to American organ transplants for well-to-do Arabians typifies this type of activity. Third party decisions to ration care may be associated with any of the other rationing mechanisms, even when entitlement and/or ability to pay criteria have been met.

2. Several authors (e.g., Caplan 1983) have questioned public acceptance and ethical concerns for tax financed replacement of cirrhotic livers among alcoholics.

3. The medical facts and figures in the next three paragraphs are largely taken from Smeeding and Straub 1984.

4. While a majority of elderly poor are income eligible for Medicaid, many have assets in excess of the Medicaid limitation. Were large medical bills to arise, most of these persons would spend down these assets to become Medicaid eligible.

5. However, between 1985 and 2010, due to a relatively slow growth in new elderly beneficiaries, the Old-Age and Survivors Disability Insurance trust fund is expected to have a surplus as high as 20 percent of GNP (Munnell 1985). Should such a situation materialize, it may be difficult to restrain Congress from adding the elderly entitlements, e.g., universal Medicare financed long-term care.

6. Such a plan has recently been introduced in the House of Representatives by Representative Stark, but details of his plan have not yet reached the author.

7. The emerging American policy seems to be that middle-aged parents should take direct financial responsibility for their children while not directly supporting their parent. Rather, tax financed benefits for the elderly provide a much larger share of their income resources than those of children.

Epilogue

Medical-Care Rationing Among the Aged: A Summary and Assessment

John P. Bunker
Bruce M. Landesman

SEVEN MAJOR THEMES or issues are raised in this volume. First, there are changing trends in mortality and longevity; people are living longer. In this century, early deaths from infectious and parasitic diseases have been replaced by later deaths from degenerative diseases. But will those who live longer be healthier? Will longer life be accompanied by improved quality, or will the years of illness and degeneration simply be increased, along with the numbers of people in declining health? There are some who argue that people will not only live longer but will be healthier, that both mortality and morbidity will be "compressed" into advanced ages. But others fear that such declines in morbidity are not likely. While this issue is debated by sociologists and statisticians, we will need to face the strong possibility that the health care needs of the elderly will not decrease; rather, an increased number of older people will need even longer periods of treatment.

Given an increasing need for health care among the elderly, the second major theme is whether or not we could afford to meet our most important health care needs, including those of the elderly, if we used our medical resources efficiently. Some contend that there is enormous waste and a serious overutilization of medical resources in our system; that we could do almost anything we want, including providing maximum life support and artificial hearts, if we put a stop to waste. In this regard, it is helpful to raise the question of the importance of involving patients in the medical decision process. Most medical care, even for the elderly, is for elective conditions in which personal values can and should play the dominant role. The paternalistic attitude of physicians may lead to widespread overtreatment of the elderly in order to provide the highest possible level of treatment, and to refrain from using procedures only when they will do certain harm. A more appropriate general rule may be to provide care only when careful studies have shown that it leads, with high probability, to relief of symptoms of disease or to cure. While the assertion that such measures to reduce waste would enable us to have all the health care we want are greeted by some with a fair amount of skepticism, all agree that we need much more data before we can be sure how great an effect reducing waste will have. In the meantime, we must be ready for the possibility that we cannot have everything we want, and that some form of health care rationing is inevitable.

With regard to the question of using resources efficiently and equitably, it is important to consider Medicare funding. Timothy M. Smeeding argues that Medicare could provide better coverage for more health needs if ineffective care were omitted, and costs spread more equitably. On the former point, he holds that Medicare should not cover organ transplants or implants until they have been shown to be effective, nor should Medicare be extended to nursing homes until subsidies for home care receive further study. On the latter point, he holds that many of the elderly are reasonably well off and can pay a larger share of their insurance premiums and costs, and more of the costs of custodial care might be borne by their children. On a different note, it was also suggested that we might do a better job in promoting cost-effective care if we put more emphasis than we do on the prevention of disease and the promotion of healthy lifestyles. Even the elderly can benefit from preventive measures. Prevention, however, will not necessarily decrease costs. It enables people to live longer, requiring more retirement benefits as well as care for the treatment of health problems later in life.

The third theme is the question of the means used to provide effective health care for the elderly, indeed for everyone. What are the mechanisms, the institutions, the procedures that can assure this? We have new health care institutions, new kinds of insurance and health plans, more competition, a greater role for the private sector, and more government regulation. Will these improve our ability to provide cost-effective care and equitable access to care for the elderly? Or will they, instead, produce age discrimination, since the elderly are the easiest targets for rationing?

A fourth and related theme is the impact of cost-consciousness on the quality of care, on the family, and on the physician-patient relationship. Worries are expressed that rationing and cost-cutting decisions will short circuit the role of the family, depersonalize the physician-patient relationship, and promote attention to budgets rather than to patient needs. We need to keep firmly in mind two levels of decision-making: the setting of public and institutional policy, and the treatment of particular patients. The demands of the former should not be allowed to dehumanize the latter.

A fifth theme is the use of various categories as modes of classification for deciding when people should and should not be eligible for care. This is particularly troubling when age cutoffs are used to decide that people will not receive care beyond a certain age, or must retire at a certain point. The troubling thing about these categories is that there is tremendous variation among the elderly in their abilities and in their quality of life. It is generally thought, for example, that memory diminishes with age. While there is some tendency in this direction, it is dependent on circumstances and can be counteracted. Further, there is great variability—some proportion of older adults perform as well at advanced ages as the best younger adults. There is a worry, then, that the use of age cutoffs is a form of age discrimination.

Another aspect of this issue concerns the decision of when to prolong life. In their study, Windt and Collette argue that decisions on these matters by the elderly and their children diverge in significant ways and depend on such factors as current life satisfaction, experience with dying, and the perceived threat to life quality. Thus, there is need for great caution in order to make decisions that truly respect the autonomous wishes of the elderly on whether or not to prolong life.

A sixth theme is the role of the public in making decisions about health care and in the rationing of such care. Several different constituencies have an interest in these decisions: physicians, health care administrators, government regulators, patients, and citizens. In this regard, it is interesting to look at the British system, which is less costly and which denies care to some categories of people who would be able to get care in this country. Francis and Francis argue that rationing decisions in Britain have not been made through the democratic political process. Rather, they have been made over time by bureaucrats and physicians. The public, however, does not know very much about these matters. British patients, it appears, have often been told that nothing further can be done for them when the truth of the matter is that something can be done, but it has not been funded. It is hard to justify the implementation of such an important social policy in a democratic political system without adequate public debate. We need to carefully consider the appropriate roles of experts, bureaucrats, and citizens in making the difficult choices facing us.

The seventh issue is the question of a time to die. Governor Lamm doubts that it is sensible to use very expensive technology to prolong a life of pain and degeneration for only a short time. Not providing such care is probably the most obvious form of rationing health care for the elderly. But Margaret Battin's paper raises questions about the implications of withholding care. When it is no longer sensible to use extraordinary measures to keep people alive, people do not die instantly. Rather, they linger on, and it is still expensive to provide them with even minimal, palliative care. If, therefore, our motive in thinking that there is a time to die is that we want to save resources that can be better used for other purposes, then perhaps we ought to end life rather than merely allow people to die. Direct termination or the encouragement of suicide, when the time to die has come, can both end suffering and lead to a more effective allocation of resources. The view that bringing about death directly is morally permissible causes much discomfort, but shows the necessity of thinking through the logical implications of believing that, at some point, we should stop providing people with medical care and let them die.

In sum, the major issues of this volume and the conference on which it is based are the problems posed by increasing life and illness, and the increasing costs of health care. How do we provide effective and nonwasteful care while avoiding lower quality, age discrimination, undemocratic decision-making, inequitable access, and other threats to our moral values. Can we ration—if we must—sensibly, morally, and justly? And, if so, how?

Index

Contributors

A. Brian Ault received a masters degree in sociology at the University of Utah in 1985. His chapter in this volume was completed while he was a graduate student at Utah. Mr. Ault is currently a research assistant at Child Trends, Inc., in Washington, D.C.

Margaret P.Battin, Associate Professor of Philosophy at the University of Utah, holds a Ph.D. from the University of California at Irvine. She is the author of *Ethical Issues in Suicide,* and an editor or co-editor of several other volumes on issues on euthanasia and suicide. She has served as philosopher-in-residence at a Veterans Administration Medical Center. She also publishes short fiction, including "Terminal Procedure," included in the Best American Short Stories of 1976, and is currently president of the Pacific Division of the American Society for Aesthetics.

John P. Bunker, M.D., is a faculty member in the Division of Health Services Research at Stanford University. He has written widely on cost-effective medical practice and variations in practical patterns for such varied forums as the *New York Review of Books* and the *New England Journal of Medicine.* Among his many books and monographs are *Costs, Risks and Benefits of Surgery,* and *The Artificial Heart: Costs, Risks and Benefits.* During 1985, he was a fellow at the Center for Advanced Study in the Behavioral Sciences at Stanford.

John Collette is Associate Professor of Sociology at the University of Utah. He has also taught and conducted research in Australia and New Zealand. His current research interests are in aging, medical sociology, and survey research. He has published several articles on aging, mental health, and gender in leading sociology and gerontology journals.

Suzanne Dandoy, M.D., received her undergraduate, medical, and public health training in epidemiology at the University of California at Los Angeles. She has held academic positions with the University of California at Los Angeles and Arizona State University, and spent two years with the Peace Corps in Ethiopia. Dr. Dandoy spent ten years in the Arizona Department of Health Services, five as director of that department. She is currently Executive Director of the Utah Department of Health.

John Francis is Associate Professor and Chairman of the Department of Political Science at the University of Utah. He has published papers on British politics, on political parties, and on public land policy, and, with Richard Ganzel, is editor of *Western Public Lands*.

Leslie P. Francis is Associate Professor of Law and Associate Professor of Philosophy at the University of Utah. She has published papers on distributive justice, on age discrimination in health care, and on a number of other issues in ethics and the philosophy of law. John and Leslie Francis are currently at work on a book on democratic decision-making in health policy.

Gary Gillund is Assistant Professor of Psychology at the University of Utah. His primary research interests are in the areas of memory performance and theoretical models of memory. An article presenting a theory of memory performance has been published in *Psychological Review* (1984, with Richard Shiffrin). Recently, Gillund has become interested in the changes in memory performance that occur across adulthood, and much of his current research is in this area.

John L. Horn is Professor of Psychology at the Univesity of Denver. He received his Ph.D. from the University of Illinois and has taught at the University of California-Berkeley, the University of London, and the University of Lund in Sweden. His research on adulthood changes in intellectual abilities has won several prizes in psychology and psychiatry. He is currently an editorial board member of the *Journal of Gerontology, Psychometricia*, and the *International Journal of Aging and Human Development*.

Dennis W. Jahnigen is Chief of the Geriatric Section, Veteran's Medical Center in Denver, Colorado, and Assistant Professor of Medicine, University of Colorado Health Sciences Center. He received his M.D. from Ohio State University in 1975. His main research interest is in geriatric medicine where he has recently published several articles. In December 1984, *Esquire Magazine* profiled him as one of the top 200 American leaders under age 40 for his work in geriatrics.

Richard D. Lamm is currently Governor of the State of Colorado. His opinions on health care rationing among the elderly and on ethical values in health care have been widely quoted in major medical publications, on network news programs, and on the McNeil-Lehrer Report.

Bruce M. Landesman is Associate Professor of Philosophy at the University of Utah. His major interests are political philosophy and professional ethics, and he has published several papers in those areas, including "Egalitarianism" *(Canadian Journal of Philosophy)* and "Confidentiality and the Lawyer-Client Relationship" (in David Luban ed., *The Good Lawyer: Lawyer's Roles and Lawyer's Ethics*, Rowman and Allanheld, 1984). He chaired the Second Annual Utah Conference on Ethics and Health, and has directed the philosophy department's professional ethics course program. He teaches courses in bioethics, business ethics, professional ethics, political philosophy, ethical theory, and Marxism.

James W. Nickel is Professor of Philosophy and Director of the Center for Values and Social Policy at the University of Colorado, Boulder. Previously, he held positions at the University of California at Berkeley Law School and at Wichita State University. His research interests lie in social, legal, and political philosophy. He has published extensively on these topics in several university law reviews (Columbia, Georgia, University of Southern California), the *American Philosophical Quarterly*, and *Philosophy and Public Affairs.*

S. Jay Olshansky received a Ph.D. in sociology from the University of Chicago where he was trained as a demographer with expertise in mortality and social epidemiology. His research and publications are in the areas of modeling mortality change and epidemiologic transitions, and have appeared in such journals as *Demography* and the *American Journal of Public Health.* He is currently working as an environmental scientist at Argonne National Laboratory.

Timothy M. Smeeding is Professor of Economics and Director of the Division of Social Science Research at the University of Utah. He has published widely on health care financing issues in the *Milbank Memorial Fund Quarterly, Health and Society,* and the *Journal of Health Politics, Policy and Law.* He is a nationally recognized authority on the income value of Medicare, Medicaid, and employer-provided health benefits, having written several articles and monographs, and having several times presented congressional testimony on this issue.

Daniel Wikler, whose Ph.D. in philosophy is from the University of California at Los Angeles, teaches in the medical ethics program at the University of Wisconsin Center for Health Sciences. He has been a member of the President's Commission for the Study of Ethical Problems in Medicine and Biomedical and Behavioral Research, and has published papers on numerous topics including brain death, paternalism, and mental retardation in several bioethics and philosophy journals.

Peter Windt is Associate Professor of Philosophy at the University of Utah. He began to specialize in bioethics in 1975, with the aid of a grant from the National Endowment for the Humanities and a fellowship from the Rockefeller Foundation. Since then, he has regularly taught courses in bioethics, and has presented many addresses, seminars, and workshops to health care professionals in a variety of fields. His current research interests include an investigation of the relationship between theoretical work in ethics, and practical decision-making and policy; a critical study of the concept of quality of life and its role in medical ethics; and a critical study of the concept of a person and the role of that concept in medical ethics.